THE SCIENCE AND PHYSIOLOGY OF FLEXIBILITY AND STRETCHING

Stretching is a fundamentally important part of sport and exercise, playing a role in improving performance, and preventing injury and rehabilitation, but its scientific underpinnings have, to this point, been overlooked in book publishing. *The Science and Physiology of Flexibility and Stretching* is the most up-to-date and comprehensive book to cover the underlying physiology and psychology of stretching, critically assessing why, when, and how we should stretch, as well as offering a highly illustrated, practical guide to stretching exercises.

Placing stretching in the context of both health and performance, the first section of the book sets out the science behind stretching, critically assessing the benefits, disadvantages, and roles of different types of stretching, exploring the mechanisms behind increasing range-of-movement through stretching and other methods, and offering evidence-based guidance on building stretching into warm-ups. In its second section, the book provides a step-by-step guide to static, dynamic, and PNF stretching exercises for beginners, through recreational athletes, to elite performers.

Richly illustrated, and including an online resource, *The Science and Physiology of Flexibility and Stretching* provides an important scientific enquiry into stretching, and an invaluable reference for any strength and conditioning coach or student, personal trainer, sports coach or exercise scientist.

David G. Behm, PhD, is a University Research Professor at the School of Human Kinetics and Recreation, Memorial University of Newfoundland, Canada. He was a highly competitive athlete, was drafted into the Canadian Football League (1979) and won Canadian provincial championships in tennis (Saskatchewan: 1987) and squash (Newfoundland: 2000, 2002). His athletic background led him to an academic career in the areas of applied neuromuscular physiology and sport/exercise science. Dr Behm has won a number of university, national, and international awards. He has published over 230 peer-reviewed scientific articles with over 14,000 citations. He consistently presents his research findings internationally and his work is often featured in popular fitness and health magazines, and online publications. He has been ranked no. 1 expert/scientist in the world for stretching by Expertscape, and no. 8 for resistance training, no. 14 for plyometrics, and no. 24 for muscle fatigue.

THE SCIENCE AND PHYSIOLOGY OF FLEXIBILITY AND STRETCHING

Implications and Applications in Sport Performance and Health

David G. Behm

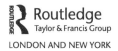

Routledge
Taylor & Francis Group

LONDON AND NEW YORK

First published 2019
by Routledge
2 Park Square, Milton Park, Abingdon, Oxon OX14 4RN

and by Routledge
711 Third Avenue, New York, NY 10017

Routledge is an imprint of the Taylor & Francis Group, an informa business

British Library Cataloguing-in-Publication Data
A catalogue record for this book is available from the British Library

Library of Congress Cataloging-in-Publication Data
Names: Behm, David G., author.
Title: The science and physiology of flexibility and stretching : implications
and applications in sport performance and health / David G. Behm.
Description: Abingdon, Oxon ; New York, NY : Routledge, 2019. |
Includes bibliographical references and index.
Identifiers: LCCN 2018023146| ISBN 9781138086906 (hbk) | ISBN
9781138086913 (pbk) | ISBN 9781315110745 (ebk)
Subjects: LCSH: Stretch (Physiology) | Stretching exercises.
Classification: LCC QP310.S77 B45 2019 | DDC 613.7/182–dc23
LC record available at https://lccn.loc.gov/2018023146

ISBN: 978-1-138-08690-6 (hbk)
ISBN: 978-1-138-08691-3 (pbk)
ISBN: 978-1-315-11074-5 (ebk)

Typeset in Bembo
by Swales & Willis Ltd, Exeter, Devon, UK

Visit the eResources: www.routledge.com/9781138086913

I dedicate this book to:

- My lovely wife, Joanne and wonderful daughter Anna, who have kept me balanced and grounded;
- My many graduate students without whom it would have been impossible to collect and disseminate such a body of sport and exercise science literature and knowledge.
- My friends and colleagues at Memorial University and around the world who continue to inspire and support me.

CONTENTS

FIGURES

TABLES

ABBREVIATIONS

5BX	5 Basic eXercises
BCE	before the common era
CE	common era
CFL	Canadian Football League
CNS	central nervous system
CR	contract relax
CRAC	contract–relax agonist–contract
DNA	deoxyribonucleic acid
DNIC	diffuse noxious inhibitory control
DOMS	delayed onset muscle soreness
E–C	excitation–contraction
EIMD	exercise-induced muscle damage
EMD	electromechanical delay
EMG	electromyography
E-reflex	exteroceptive reflex
GTO	Golgi tendon organ
HPA	hypothalamic–pituitary–adrenal
H-reflex	Hoffman reflex
Hz	Hertz
ICC	intraclass correlation coefficient
MEP	motor-evoked potential
MGF	mechano-growth factor
MMG	mechanomyogram
MTU	musculotendinous unit
MVC	maximal voluntary contraction
M-wave	muscle action potential wave
PIC	persistent inward currents

PNF	proprioceptive neuromuscular facilitation
RCMP	Royal Canadian Mounted Police
ROM	range of motion
SEBT	Star Excursion Balance Test
SSC	stretch-shortening cycle
TMS	transcranial magnetic stimulation
T-reflex	tendon reflex
XBX	10 basic exercises

1

MY PERSONAL MOTIVATION FOR STRETCHING

The year is 1972. A 15-year-old, 5 foot 10 inch (1.78 metres), 175 lb (79.4 kg) fullback takes his stance 3 yards behind the quarterback. This grade 11 fullback playing junior high school football is bigger and stronger than most of the offensive linemen blocking for him as well as most of the young adolescent opponents who will try to tackle him. With the ball snapped on the second "hut", the quarterback rotates and hands the ball off to the fullback who is accelerating to an expected opening between the tight end and tackle. As the tight end cross blocks upon the defensive end and the offensive tackle pulls out against the linebacker, a sliver of daylight appears. I lower my shoulder and plunge through that hole. Arms reach out from the partially blocked defensive lineman and linebacker but they are not strong enough to slow me down. A strong side defensive back at about 140 lb (63.5 kg) moves in for the tackle. However, with the momentum of my greater mass and the velocity attained after an 8-yard sprint, the defensive back is trampled and I cut sharply to the sidelines. After covering about 20 yards, the defensive safety catches me from behind and trips me up.

The next year, I am the starting fullback for the senior high school team. I have grown ¾ inch (2 cm) and now weigh 185 lb (84 kg). We win the regional high school championship. Dave Behm (The Truck) and Dan (Crazy Legs) Murphy make a great 1–2 punch. My predominant empire is between the two ends. Dives and off-tackle plays are my bread and butter. If I get a decent block and get into the defensive backfield, I can use my size advantage, my balance, and my signature move: hit the opponent at full throttle to either knock him down or spin immediately after contact so that the enemy cannot easily grab me and pull me down. Murphy's territory is outside the ends with sweeps and pitches because he is lighter and much swifter than I and can often outsprint the defence.

In the last year of high school, there is no increase in height but I continue to fill out, expanding to 198 lb (90 kg). A number of Canadian universities attempt to recruit me and I decide to stay home to play with the University of Ottawa Gee-Gees, who had lost that year in the national semi-final game. However, as the next year approaches, I realize that my chances of getting into a game with that team are slim to none. The starting fullback is Neil Lumsden, a 235 lb (106 kg) behemoth with decent speed, great balance, strength, and power. He will set Canadian university rushing and touchdown records that will remain untouched for a couple of decades and he will subsequently establish a long career in the professional Canadian Football League (CFL). The back-up is Mike Murphy, another talented fullback at just under 230 lb (104 kg) who in the following year will lead the nation in rushing yards and also have a firm career in the CFL. I decide to play for the city's junior football team (Ottawa Sooners) and wait for Lumsden to move on to the CFL. Lumsden and Murphy were archetype fullbacks, massive, strong, and powerful. Relatively, I filled that description in high school but my growth pattern started to plateau, such that I was around 205 lb (93 kg) when I joined the university football team in my second year of university. I spent my second year of university primarily blocking for the burly Mike Murphy and moved into the fullback position in my third academic year. I was lucky enough to inherit a strong offensive line and with my slashing, spinning style I could often break a few tackles and make a major gain (Figure 1.1). With my lack of breakaway running speed, I was typically caught from behind by a fleet-footed defensive back. For a professional running back,

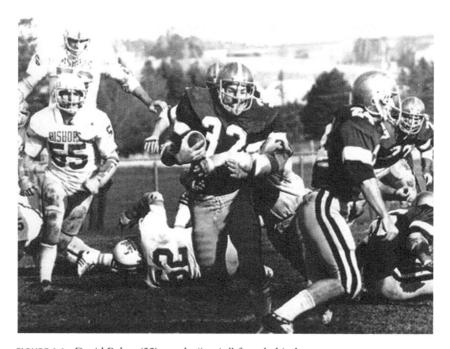

FIGURE 1.1 David Behm (32) caught "again" from behind

my size was more typical of tailbacks or halfbacks, depending on your terminology. These backs typified by legends such as Walter Payton had very good to great speed that would allow them to burst into the open field and outsprint the opposition. Unfortunately, I was built like a tailback but with the speed of a fullback. I needed to get faster if I wanted to continue my career after university.

Sprinting speed is a simple combination of stride rate (frequency) and stride length (1). Stride rate is very difficult to modify because it is generally related to your genetic profile of fast-twitch to slow-twitch muscle fibre composition. Pick the right parents, who hopefully will pass on a higher percentage of fast-twitch fibres and you will be able to move your legs back and forth (stride rate) much quicker than someone with a greater percentage of slow-twitch fibres. Hence, you will have a high stride rate. This is the most important factor in sprinting speed. Unfortunately, it seems that I did not pick the right parents! Thus, I was left with trying to enhance the second sprinting factor: stride length. With stronger, more powerful legs, it should be possible to explode off the ground and cover greater distances with each stride. With this in mind, I worked faithfully on my strength, such that I could squat over 500 lb (225 kg) and bench press around 350 lb (160 kg). As a university student in physical education in the late 1970s, I was taught that by increasing my flexibility I would improve performance (increase stride length, decrease resistance to stride movements) and decrease the chances of injury.

With these pearls of wisdom in mind, I also worked diligently on my stretching so that I could eventually perform a front split. Conventional wisdom of the time indicated that with higher levels of flexibility there would be less resistance to movement and an increased efficiency of movement. Thus, with my improved power and flexibility my stride length should have been tremendous. Like Superman, I should have been leaping over tall buildings in a single bound. However, there must have been some kryptonite in my diet because, while my sprinting speed did improve marginally, nobody ever mistook me for the legendary Walter Payton (or Superman!).

Well if I did not get much faster, then my flexibility should have decreased my chances for injury. In my second year of university football, I took the ball on a draw play (quarterback fakes a pass and then gives the ball to the running back) and burst through a gap in the line. Quickly a linebacker exploded from the left accelerating his helmet into my shoulder. I tried to absorb the hit and I bounced off the hit and continued for another 12 yards till I was, as usual, caught from behind by a defensive back. On getting up I noticed my clavicle was apparently redirected towards my back and no longer attached to my scapula. When I returned to the sidelines I was informed that I had subluxated my acromioclavicular joint. I was out for the season.

With aggressive rehabilitation and off-season training I was ready for my third year of university football. In a game against McGill University on artificial turf, I caught a flare pass and sprinted wide. As I planted my right foot to move up field I was hit low on the left side by a linebacker and simultaneously hit high from the right by a defensive back. My planted foot could not move or slide on the artificial turf and the ligaments were torn resulting in a third-degree ankle sprain. It did not seem that my extensive stretching programme had provided me the protection I sought from musculotendinous or ligamentous injuries nor did it provide me with significantly better athletic performance (improved speed). Did my physical education professors of the 1970s really know what they were talking about? The paradigm of stretching and flexibility has experienced a number of shifts in the past few decades and hopefully this book will help establish the facts as they are presently known, and burst the myths.

It is the objective of this book to provide you with the most up-to-date research on stretching and flexibility by explaining the physiological mechanisms underlying different types of stretching and flexibility exercises, and then provide you with suggestions for appropriate activity programmes to increase your range of motion.

Reference

1. Dintiman G and Ward B. *Sport Speed*. Windsor, ON: Human Kinetics Publishers, 2003.

2

HISTORY OF STRETCHING

Stretching has been and continues to be a controversial training technique. When did it begin? Is it actually beneficial? Often, I have heard individuals state that, if stretching was important for performance enhancement, you would see lions, tigers, and cheetahs meeting in groups (wearing spandex and knee braces) for a stretching routine before going on a hunt. Although our mammalian cousins are not quite that organized, we do see animals stretching after sleeping or lounging for an extended period of time. This ritualized behaviour is called pandiculation, and involves a voluntary contraction of the muscles, followed by a slow stretch/elongation and then relaxation (often with a yawn) (Figure 2.1). The description is somewhat similar to contract–relax PNF (without the yawn), which was reported to be developed by Herman Kabat, but perhaps he stole the idea from his pet dog or cat (if he had a pet?). One simply has to watch a pet dog or cat to see them stretching their fore and hind limbs after napping. Animals stretch (pandiculate) all the time! Is it a reflex ritual that actually benefits performance (hunting prey or escaping from predators)? Lions and tigers are not very accessible or easy subjects to recruit and I do not know of any stretch-training studies using domesticated pets. Thus, there is no evidence for or against the effectiveness of pandiculation for performance enhancement. Obviously, animals (other than the human animal) have not organized and categorized their stretching and warm-up activities as humans have. Nor do animals stretch for such long durations or intensely as many human athletes or trained individuals. Of course, they also do not play tennis for 3–4 hours like professional tennis players, crash into each other for more than an hour like American football, rugby, and ice hockey players, or perform *multiple* double or triple rotations of their bodies with twists for over 1–3 minutes like gymnasts, dancers, figure skaters, trampolinists, and others. Other mammals can be far more athletic than humans, but they tend to perform their athletic pursuits as a prey or a predator over a brief period, sporadically, and

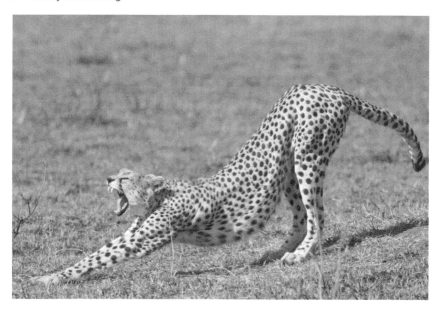

FIGURE 2.1 Pandiculation

without hours of training per day over months and years. We as humans tend to be far more obsessive and compulsive in our activities, and likewise in our training for those activities. There is a common assumption that animals never get injured. There is no evidence for this assumption. Racehorses, for example, commonly sustain muscle strains and have a high incidence of tendinopathy (1). Dogs suffer strains (muscles) and sprains (ligaments) (2). So maybe if they had better warm-up and stretching routines, they would experience fewer injuries? It is also argued that animals and ourselves often sprint without any warm-up (e.g. we are late for a bus!) and many times either catch the prey, escape from the predator, or actually catch the bus. Thus, the contrarians argue there is no need for a warm-up. The problem with this argument is there is no control group! Nobody has taken a pride of lions and systematically stretched them over time and compared their performance with a control group of lions that did not stretch or only pandiculated. Perhaps, the lion would be incrementally faster if it did do a systematic warm-up. Although there is no evidence available for wild predators and prey, there is a large body of human research available about positive changes to neural conduction velocity, enzymatic cycling, tissue compliance, and a myriad of other contributing physiological factors. We will cover many of these topics in subsequent chapters.

When did humans start stretching in an organized manner with the hope of enhancing performance or decreasing the chance for injury? Although, in historical texts, stretching is not always precisely listed as an activity preceding training or competition, it might be logical to assume that military personnel or athletes would have indulged in some kind of "limbering up" exercises to warm the muscles and body and increase the compliance or decrease the stiffness of the muscle and tendons. The martial arts of many Asian countries are well known for their emphasis on extreme range of motion (ROM) in order to perform high kicks, and acrobatic and escape manoeuvres (think of Bruce Lee's athletic ability). The martial arts of the Chinese, Japanese, and Aleut peoples, as well as Mongolian wrestling, are suggested to have originated in the prehistoric era (3). Chinese boxing has been traced to the Zhou dynasty (1122–255 BCE). Martial arts like Kung Fu were influenced by Indian martial arts which spread to China in the fifth to sixth century CE (3). With the physical contortions, commonly observed with wrestling and martial arts, it would seem likely that the combatants would have needed to work on their flexibility to improve their chances of succeeding.

We are all familiar with the impressive flexibility of experienced yoga practitioners as they move from one difficult posture to another. Asia and specifically the Indus–Sarasvati civilization in northern India are credited with the origins of Yoga during what is termed the "pre-classical yoga period" approximately 5000 years ago and perhaps even earlier. However, this early yoga practice concentrated on the mind and spirit with little to no emphasis on the physical. Breath control exercises, the precursor of yoga, were implemented in China around 2600 BCE. It is not known if stretching exercises were also included but an exercise chart (168 BCE) of breathing and postures was developed for Tao Yin activities in the early Han dynasty. These exercises or postures were purported to cure specific illnesses (4). Perhaps, this is where the idea that stretching decreases injuries first began. Around the fourth century, during what is classified as the post-classical Yoga (classical Yoga period defined by Patanjali's Yoga-Sûtras "eight limbed path" to Samadhi or enlightenment starting in the second century CE), a system of practices was created to rejuvenate the body, prolong life, and embrace the physical body to achieve enlightenment. Tantra Yoga was developed to cleanse the body and mind. The evolution of these physical–spiritual connections and body-centred practices moved towards the development of Hatha Yoga (Figure 2.2).

Stretching is specifically mentioned as an important component of an exercise regimen to prevent illness by Hua Tuo (104–208 CE). Hua Tuo suggested mimicking animal movements such as walking like a bear, and stretching the neck like a bird (even 2000 years ago people noticed that animals stretched or at least pandiculated), among other animal-like movements. He emphasized combinations of breathing, bending, stretching, and an assortment of postures that he labelled the "Frolics of the Five Animals" (4). Tai Chi may trace its beginnings to these frolicking exercises.

In the western civilizations, the Greeks held festivals (Tailteann Games: circa 1800 BCE) that involved stone throwing, jumping, spear throwing, wrestling, and other activities (4). During pharaonic Egyptian times, athletes also wrestled, boxed, swam, ran, and lifted heavy objects in competition. One can imagine that these athletes had some kind of pre-competition preparation (warm-up) and

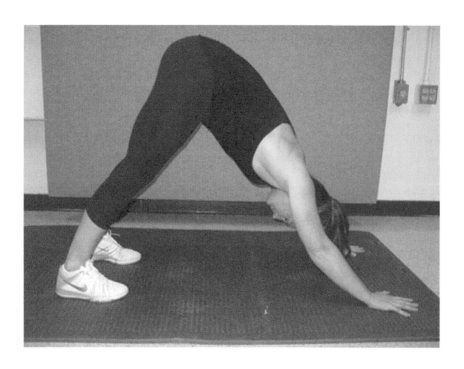

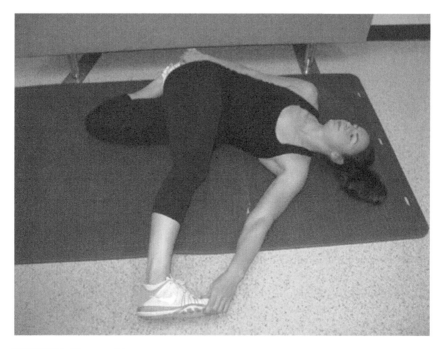

FIGURE 2.2 Yoga positions

that, especially for sports like wrestling where limbs can be forced and placed in extreme positions, preparatory stretching would have taken place. Were these early stretching exercises more static or dynamic in nature?

First of all, how do we define static and dynamic stretching? Static stretching involves lengthening a muscle until either a stretch sensation or the point of discomfort is reached and then holding the muscle in a lengthened position for a prescribed period of time (5–7). Dynamic stretching involves the performance of a controlled movement through the ROM of the active joint(s) (6,7). Both types of stretching have gone through periods of popularity and disfavour. For example, Hua Tuo's stretching the neck like a bird exercise would likely have involved a slow dynamic component to reach the end of the ROM and then a static component to hold that position. Dynamic stretching was popular in Persia where warriors and wrestlers, starting around the first century AD, used implements shaped like bowling pins called meels (Figure 2.3). Although the heavy meels weighed approximately 50 lb and would have been used for strength and power enhancement, the 2-lb meels were swung in patterns around the shoulder and would have been excellent for a dynamic warm-up of the muscles and increasing the ROM. The Persians introduced this form of exercise to the Indian subcontinent in the thirteenth century. The people of the India subcontinent called this activity Persian yoga (4). It is quite likely that similar movement variations with a variety of weapons (i.e. short and long swords) would have been practiced by medieval knights in preparation for combat and competitions.

Generally, such light dynamic movement for flexibility, quickness, and muscular endurance was in the purview of men getting ready for battles or tournaments.

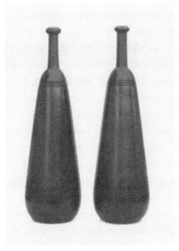

Meel

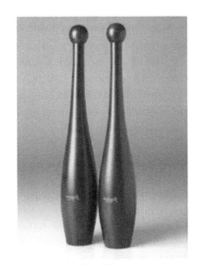

Indian Clubs

FIGURE 2.3 Persian meels and Indian clubs

However, in the mid-nineteenth century, exercises based on Swedish (Ling's) gymnastics were introduced to women in Europe and North America. They involved the graceful moving of arms, legs, neck, and head. Although their primary purpose (training for family life) would not have been to increase flexibility, such movements would have maintained or enhanced movement around the exercised joints. These "exercise-liberated" women could now be more effective at reaching farther across to make the bed in the mornings, extending further to scrub the floor under the furniture, or reach deeper in the cupboard for the pots and pans for making dinner (training for family life!). Quite the liberation! Men, on the other hand, would still incorporate low-intensity or light dynamic movements for sport preparation or war.

The late nineteenth century saw the emergence of a number of new team sports such as ice hockey (3 March 1875: Montreal, Quebec, Canada), baseball (1672–1700: England), basketball (1891 by James Naismith [Canadian] at Springfield College, Massachusetts, USA), North American football (6 November 1869, Rutgers vs Princeton University, USA), volleyball (1895 by William G. Morgan from Springfield College, Massachusetts, USA), and others. The typical competitive zeal of the human athlete would instil a need to find a perceived advantage even in the early days of these new sports. One of those advantages could be a proper warm-up to prepare the body for competition and part of that warm-up would include light dynamic movements for "limbering up".

But more importantly was the defence of your country and, during the World Wars, soldiers were systematically trained to ensure that they were ready for heavy military action. The systematic training of soldiers was incorporated during the World Wars with scientific investigations of optimal resistance training routines sought out by Colonel DeLorme of the US armed forces (8,9). Subsequently, in the late 1950s and published in 1961, a Canadian, Dr William Orban, developed the 5BX (5 Basic eXercises) programme. Although it was originally targeted at male military personnel (air force pilots) who might not have access to training equipment, and thus could perform calisthenics in almost any location to stay fit, it spread to the general population. Orban also developed the XBX which were 10 basic exercises modified for women. One of the stated objectives was to: "Keep the important muscles and joints of the body supple and flexible." Some of the exercises were quite dynamic and ballistic such as the toe-touching exercises, which involved bobbing up and down by flexing at the hips to touch the toes, and then bouncing back to an erect standing position.

However, the appeal of dynamic ballistic stretching activities diminished when it was noted that dynamic stretching of the muscles activated reflexes such as the myotactic (i.e. stretch) reflex, which results in reflexive contractions of the actively stretched muscle (10,11). If the goal of stretching was to increase the ROM, then it was reasoned that dynamic activities that elicited reflex muscle contractions while elongating the muscles could result in injury. Two forces would be working against each other with muscle elongation from stretching opposing stretch reflex-induced contractions. Hence, during the mid-1960s and thereafter, static stretching replaced ballistic or dynamic stretching as the predominant activity within a pre-activity warm-up routine to increase the ROM (12,13). Static stretching was recommended because the slow movement into the stretch position and maintenance of a static stretch over a prolonged period minimized the reflexive firing of the muscle spindles that were activated by higher rates of stretch (14,15). Hence, the attenuation of reflex activity with prolonged static stretching would presumably result in a more relaxed muscle and theoretically allow greater muscle lengths to be achieved. Thus, for the next 30+ years, static stretching was the predominant form of stretching for warm-ups and flexibility.

In the 1970s, another stretching technique also became more popular: proprioceptive neuromuscular facilitation (PNF) stretching. PNF was developed around 1946 by Herman Kabat, a neurophysiologist. The techniques evolved over time, but one popular variation of PNF was the contract relax–agonist contract (CRAC) method. If you wanted to stretch the hamstrings you would **contract** the hip flexors (i.e. quadriceps) till you reached your maximum ROM. Then you would **relax** as your partner held that elongated position, which would be followed by **contraction** of the hamstrings (**agonists**). These variations of PNF were purported to induce a number of inhibitory reflex mechanisms (e.g. reciprocal inhibition, autogenic inhibition) that would relax the muscle, allowing the individual to reach even greater increases in ROM than with static stretching. You could not go to any team sport in the 1970s without seeing athletes pairing up to passively stretch and provide resistance to their partner's contractions of elongated muscles. However, not many people questioned, at the time, why a technique like PNF which supposedly inhibited excitatory reflexes would be used in a warm-up that should excite the system in preparation for high-intensity activity.

In the late 1990s and early 2000s, scientific reports began to appear indicating that static stretching rather than enhancing subsequent performance might actually impair performance. As the evidence began to mount throughout the early twenty-first century, static stretching was replaced with dynamic stretching as the major flexibility component of the warm-up. Only recently has the evidence for static stretch-induced performance impairments been suggested to lack some ecological validity (practical reality or real-life application). A position stand/review by the Canadian Society for Exercise Physiology (6), published in 2016, documented that many of the static stretching studies did not employ a prior aerobic-style warm-up, stretched the muscle(s) for durations much longer than are typically used, did not include any dynamic sport specific activities after stretching, and conducted the testing within 3–4 minutes of the experimental protocol. Another study found that just knowledge of the previously published stretching-impairment studies (expectancy bias) could negatively affect the results (16). Thus, the state of stretching within a warm-up and for improving ROM is in a state of flux and confusion. The objective of this book is to alleviate some of that confusion by critically analysing the 5Ws of stretching with an "H" thrown in for good measure, i.e.

1. **What** are the effects and physiological mechanisms underlying different types of stretching?
2. **Why** should we stretch?
3. **When** should we stretch?
4. **Who** are the major pioneers, innovators, and researchers in this area?
5. **Where** does the science of flexibility and stretching go next?
6. **How** should we stretch or use other techniques to increase ROM?

Summary

Many animals elongate (stretch) their muscles after a period of rest. Although, these animals have pandiculated for eons, it is not known whether there are any performance benefits. There is inferential evidence that humans have stretched for thousands of years with the advent of yoga (~3000 BCE) and martial arts (~1000 BCE) in Asia. The Greeks and Egyptians probably emphasized dynamic actions and stretches before their athletic competitions (~2000 BCE). Static stretching became more popular after the World Wars, whereas PNF stretching was popularized to a greater degree in the 1970s. Both stretching styles remained predominant until the 1990s, when research began to appear indicating that static stretching could lead to performance impairments. Since that time dynamic stretching has made a resurgence. The most recent studies suggest that the move away from static stretching may have been premature and based on impractical study designs.

References

1. Parkin TD. Epidemiology of racetrack injuries in racehorses. *Vet Clin North Am Equine Pract* 24: 1–19, 2008.
2. Levy M, Hall C, Trentacosta N, and Percival M. A preliminary retrospective survey of injuries occurring in dogs participating in canine agility. *Vet Comp Orthop Traumatol* 22: 321–324, 2009.
3. Draeger DF and Smith RW. *Comprehensive Asian Fighting Arts*. Tokyo: Kodansha, 1969.
4. Kunitz D. *Lift: Fitness Culture from Naked Greeks and Acrobats to Jazzercize and Ninja Warriors*. New York: Harper Wave, 2016.
5. Behm DG, Bambury A, Cahill F, and Power K. Effect of acute static stretching on force, balance, reaction time, and movement time. *Med Sci Sports Exerc* 36: 1397–1402, 2004.
6. Behm DG, Blazevich AJ, Kay AD, and McHugh M. Acute effects of muscle stretching on physical performance, range of motion, and injury incidence in healthy active individuals: A systematic review. *Appl Physiol Nutr Metab* 41: 1–11, 2016.
7. Behm DG and Chaouachi A. A review of the acute effects of static and dynamic stretching on performance. *Eur J Appl Physiol* 111: 2633–2651, 2011.
8. Delorme T. Restoration of muscle power by heavy-resistance exercises. *J Bone Joint Surg* 27: 645–667, 1945.

9. Delorme T, Ferris B, and Gallagher J. Effect of progressive resistance exercise on muscle contraction time. *Arch Phys Med* 33: 86–92, 1952.

10. Matthews PBC. Developing views on the muscle spindle. In: *Spinal and Supraspinal Mechanisms of Voluntary Motor Control and Locomotion.* JE Desmedt, ed. Basel: Karger, 1980, pp. 12–27.

11. Matthews PBC. Muscle spindles: Their messages and their fusimotor supply. In: *The Nervous System: Handbook of Physiology.* VB Brooks, ed. American Physiological Society, 1981, pp. 189–288.

12. Young WB. The use of static stretching in warm-up for training and competition. *Int J Sports Physiol Perform* 2: 212–216, 2007.

13. Young WB and Behm DG. Effects of running, static stretching and practice jumps on explosive force production and jumping performance. *J Sports Med Phys Fitness* 43: 21–27, 2003.

14. Durbaba R, Taylor A, Ellaway PH, and Rawlinson S. The influence of bag2 and chain intrafusal muscle fibers on secondary spindle afferents in the cat. *J Physiol* 550: 263–278, 2003.

15. Laporte Y, Emonet-DÇF, and Jami L. The skeletofusimotor or beta-innervation of mammalian muscle spindles. In: *The Motor system in Neurobiology.* EV Evarts, SP Wise, and D Bousfield, eds. New York: Elsevier Biomedical Press, 1985, pp. 173–177.

16. Janes WC, Snow BB, Watkins CE, Noseworthy EA, Reid JC, and Behm DG. Effect of participants' static stretching knowledge or deception on the responses to prolonged stretching. *Appl Physiol Nutr Metab* 41: 1052–1056, 2016.

3

TYPES OF STRETCHING AND THE EFFECTS ON FLEXIBILITY

There are a number of different types of stretching and the public can be confused about their differences. Passive and active static stretching, dynamic, ballistic, proprioceptive neuromuscular facilitation (PNF), and other stretches are used to enhance flexibility or range of motion (ROM) as well as being incorporated as part of a pre-competition or training warm-up. First of all, what is the definition of flexibility? Michael J. Alter, in his textbook (1), lists a variety of definitions, some of which include:

1. ROM available to a joint or group of joints (2–6);
2. Total achievable excursion (within limits of pain) of a body part through its potential ROM (7);
3. Ability to move a joint smoothly and easily through its complete pain-free ROM (8,9);
4. Ability to move a joint through a normal ROM without undue stress to the musculotendinous unit (10); and
5. Normal joint and soft-tissue ROM in response to active or passive stretch (11).

The ability to increase a joint's ROM would normally necessitate an improved extensibility (12) or decreased stiffness of musculotendinous and other connective tissues. Gajdosik and colleagues (13,14) suggest that flexibility should be described as a ratio of change in muscle length or joint angle to a change in force or torque. Recent research uses this description or technique by subjecting a limb joint to an extended ROM on an isokinetic dynamometer as a test for muscle stiffness (15–19).

To achieve these increases in flexibility, a variety of stretching techniques is used. Static stretching, for example, involves lengthening a muscle until either a stretch sensation or the point of discomfort is reached, and then holding the muscle in a lengthened position for a prescribed period of time (20–23). Whether it is passive or active, static stretching depends on whether the muscle is lengthened by an external force (i.e. another person, or a tool such as a stretching band or machine) with the muscle relaxed (passive static stretch) or by an active contraction of the affected muscle or other muscles (i.e. antagonist; active static stretch) (Figure 3.1). Static stretching is used in athletic, fitness, health, and rehabilitation environments. It is an effective method for increasing joint ROM (24–26) and was purported to improve performance (27,28) and reduce the incidence of activity-related injuries (20–22,29–32). However, the possibility of static stretch-induced performance impairments has limited its use in the new millennium. Evidence for and against this bias is presented in a subsequent chapter.

Dynamic stretching uses a controlled movement through the ROM of the active joint(s) (33). It can be exemplified by swinging the legs back and forth (hip flexion and extension) or side to side (hip abduction and adduction) or swinging the arms in circles (shoulder circumduction) (Figure 3.2). Dynamic stretching differs from ballistic stretching in that the latter would typically involve higher-velocity movements with bouncing actions at the end of the ROM (34,35). Ballistic movements were used in the aforementioned 5BX programme (popular from the 1950s to the 1960s) and were still prevalent until quite recently in many

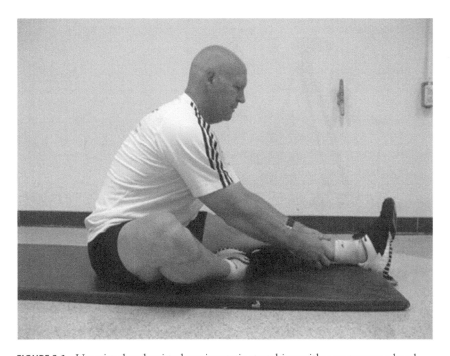

FIGURE 3.1 Unassisted and assisted passive static stretching with a partner or a band

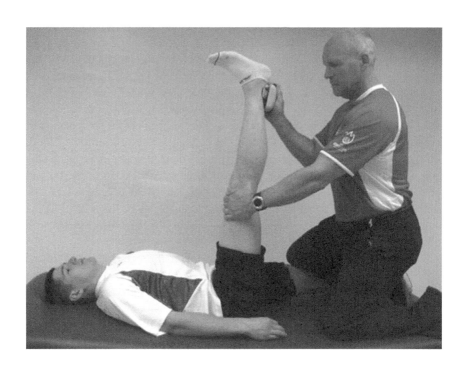

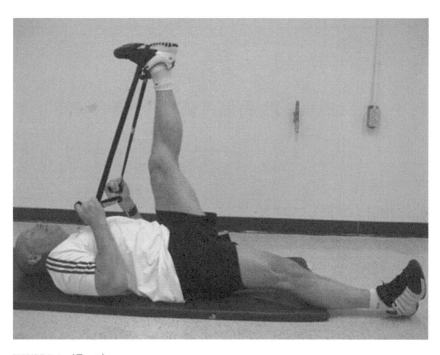

FIGURE 3.1 (Cont.)

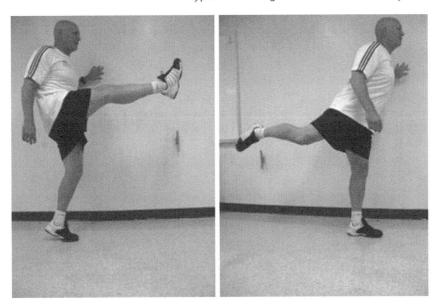

FIGURE 3.2 Dynamic stretching (hip extension and flexion)

military- and police-style training courses. In the late 1980s, I consulted with fitness instructors of The Royal Canadian Mounted Police (RCMP) at their national training depot in Regina, Saskatchewan, Canada. Recruits were trained and tested by performing resistance exercises such as shoulder presses, push-ups, sit-ups, and others as quickly as possible in a prescribed time. The number of repetitions completed in 30 or 60 seconds was measured and thus the recruits would ballistically throw the barbells up and down (i.e. shoulder press) or slam their trunk back and forth (i.e. sit-ups) as quickly as possible. Definitely a recipe for injuries!

What is the difference between dynamic stretching and dynamic activity? It could be argued that dynamic stretching is a dynamic activity but not all dynamic activities are considered to be dynamic stretching. The decisive factor is whether the dynamic activity moves the body through a full or almost full ROM. Jogging, skipping, hopping, and other similar activities are all dynamic but, as they only emphasize a restricted or small-to-moderate ROM, they would not be considered dynamic stretching. However, if the person did butt (gluteal) kicks (knee flexion, touching the buttocks with heel of the foot) while jogging, then this dynamic activity would be under the purview of dynamic stretching because it goes through a fuller ROM. As mentioned in Chapter 2, dynamic stretching in this millennium was considered preferable to static stretching in a warm-up due to training specificity (training movement matches the sport or exercise movements) (36,37), as well as activity-induced increases in metabolism, muscle temperature (27,38–40), and neural activation (41–43).

PNF stretching combines static stretching and isometric contractions in a cyclical pattern. PNF was developed in the late 1940s and early 1950s by Herman Kabat, and two physical therapists, Margaret Knott and Dorothy Voss. Kabat, was a neurophysiologist, who developed PNF based on the neuromuscular research of Sir Charles Sherrington (44,45). Two of the more ubiquitous techniques are the contract relax (CR) and contract relax agonist contract (CRAC) techniques (46,47). The CR method includes a static stretching component followed immediately by an isometric contraction of the stretched muscle, then followed with another stretch of the target muscle. CRAC involves an additional contraction of the agonist muscle (i.e. opposing the muscle group being stretched) during the stretch, before the additional stretching of the target muscle (Figure 3.3). PNF was used extensively by team athletes (PNF stretches typically need a partner) in the late twentieth century, but, similar to static stretching, its use has diminished in the twenty-first century. A number of individual studies suggest that PNF is more effective than static or dynamic stretching for improving ROM (48–50). However, a recent meta-analytic systematic review reported an advantage for static stretch training over PNF training for increasing ROM (51).

Why should we stretch? Stretching is primarily used to increase joint ROM. When used as part of a warm-up, the increased ROM was thought to improve

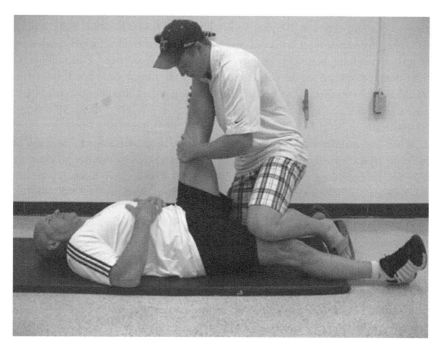

FIGURE 3.3 Proprioceptive neuromuscular facilitation (PNF) stretching for the hamstrings

performance and decrease the incidence of injuries (21,22,40). Although the ability to increase ROM through stretching is generally universally agreed, its impact on performance and injuries is more controversial. There are many factors to consider including the type, duration (volume), intensity of stretching, and the population that is stretching (i.e. male, female, young, old, athletic, sedentary, or others) among other factors. Others may use stretching to achieve a greater sense of relaxation (i.e. yoga – psychological or neurological effects).

Stretching-induced changes in range of motion

First of all, flexibility is not a global phenomenon of the body (52), i.e. an individual can be flexible in one joint but not others (52). Even within a joint they may have a greater ROM with one movement versus another. A baseball pitcher may not exhibit similar relative flexibility to a discus thrower when comparing shoulder horizontal extension versus shoulder internal and external rotation. Some joints are more susceptible to stretch-induced increases in ROM. For example, stretching the calf muscles provides only small increases in ankle dorsiflexion, which may not be clinically meaningful (53). What factors restrict our joint flexibility? Muscle fascicles (structural proteins such as myosin, actin, titin, and others), tendons, aponeuroses, joint capsules, and ligaments contribute to ROM restrictions with passive muscle elongation. As the composition of a human can range from 50% to 78% fluid (water), dependent on age, sex, hydration, and other factors, the viscosity of the tissues can substantially affect flexibility. Furthermore, a highly activated central nervous system could increase muscle tonus and with a less relaxed muscle inhibit flexibility. In addition, pushing a joint to its maximum ROM can be uncomfortable or painful, and thus the ability to tolerate this discomfort or pain may allow some individuals to stretch further than other more pain-sensitive individuals (54).

Stretching can induce elastic or plastic changes of the musculotendinous system. Elastic changes are defined as the elongation of tissues which recover when the tension has been removed; so, it is a temporary increase in ROM. Plastic changes involve a musculotendinous elongation in which the tissue deformation remains even after the tension has been removed; so, it is considered a semi-permanent change in flexibility. Elastic changes are the increases in ROM that are experienced immediately after a single session of stretching. A single session of static stretching can induce small-to-large relative ROM increases that persist for 5 (55), 10 (20,56,57), 30 (58), 90 (59), and 120 minutes (26). Evidence of persistent improved ROM even one day later has been reported (60), but not all studies show prolonged ROM increases; two 15-second passive stretches did not provide a significant improvement in ROM at any time post-stretch (61), whereas augmented ROM was only evident for 3 minutes after four 30-second static stretches (62) and only for 6 minutes after five, modified, hold-and-relax stretches (63). Specific training-induced plastic changes and mechanisms are discussed later.

As mentioned previously, there is much conflict about what type of stretching provides the greatest ROM. PNF has been reported to provide greater acute or elastic ROM improvements than static stretching in some studies (64–66), which contrasts with other studies that found similar ROM changes between PNF and static stretching (67,68). A 6-week training study reported no significant difference between static and PNF for increasing ROM, nor did either pro-gramme have any effect on drop-jump performance (69). A recent meta-analytic systematic review determined only trivial differences in ROM improvements between acute and chronic PNF and static stretching (70), whereas another review found that chronic static stretch training provided greater flexibility than PNF training (51). Dynamic stretching is also controversial, with some studies reporting that a single session of dynamic stretching provides either similar (71,72) or greater (73,74) ROM increases to static stretching. But, once again, conflicting studies report that dynamic stretching is not as effective as static stretching when used as part of a warm-up (34,75–78). Ballistic stretching (higher-velocity move-ments with bouncing actions at the end of the ROM), which can be considered a variation of dynamic stretching, was not as effective as static stretching for improving ROM after a 4-week training programme (79). When comparing static with ballistic stretching in a single (acute) stretching session, ballistic stretching has been reported to provide less ROM than static (34), or PNF (75), but a similar ROM to static stretching (SS) and PNF in another study (80). Only one study compared PNF and dynamic stretching and indicated that after 14 training sessions PNF provided 3–7% greater ROM increases (81).

Another form of stretching is termed "neuromobilization". With neuromobiliza-tion, the nerve is placed under a lengthening stress, e.g. when performing a seated straight-leg raise, the individual would actively dorsiflex the foot and flex the cervical spine to exert a type of neural traction (Figure 3.4). In an 8-week stretch training study, neuromobilization provided a greater increase in hamstring length versus PNF in the first 4 weeks but, in the last 4 weeks, hamstring length actually decreased. Thus, overall, passive static stretching provided the greatest benefits (82).

Our psychological state or emotions can affect flexibility. Two sessions, of 20 min each, of anti-anxiety techniques such as the neuro-emotional technique (also known as a mind–body technique) was shown in one study to enhance ROM to a greater extent than a similar duration of passive static stretching or no stretching (83). It is purported that latent anxiety, even if not apparent, can lead to learned emotional responses that affect the motor responses. Anti-anxiety techniques would dissipate these responses and lead to greater muscle relaxation and lower muscle tonus. Various forms of yoga combine the physical aspects of stretching with meditation or relaxation techniques to enhance the effects on flexibility.

Yoga

Serious yoga practitioners are widely known for their enhanced flexibility (84). However, yoga is also reported to improve a wide array of physiological and

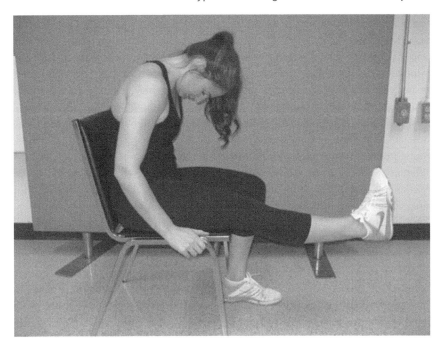

FIGURE 3.4   Neuromobilization

psychological parameters. For instance, it has been reported to increase muscular strength (85,86) and endurance (86), balance (84), maximal oxygen uptake (86), improved reaction times (85), and breath-holding times (85), reduce cardiovascular risk, blood pressure, and body mass index (87), and unify the body, mind, and spirit, among others. How can yoga stretching accomplish all these beneficial measures? Yoga misperception is the problem. Yoga is not just stretching but involves many other components. In addition to the stretching aspect, full yoga practitioners should experience changes in their mental attitude (i.e. meditation), diet, and practice of specific techniques for postures (asanas) and breathing practices (pranayamas) in order to attain a higher level of consciousness. It is unlikely that the average North American or European who goes to a trendy hot yoga session or most yoga sessions is serious or committed to a degree that they will attain a new level of consciousness. However, 30–60 min of stretching, changing positions, and holding various postures (dynamic and static muscle endurance), and inspiratory and expiratory breathing techniques will certainly enhance a variety of physiological and health parameters. From personal experience, having participated only in a single 60-minute yoga session, I experienced exercise-induced muscle soreness and delayed-onset muscle soreness for days thereafter. Although I am considered a relatively very fit individual for my age, I was not accustomed to the prolonged and slow eccentric contractions when moving from one posture to the next, or the ability to hold certain postures under extended muscle positions for prolonged periods. A lack of task specificity was certainly evident in my muscle pain over the next few days. Hence, you should not directly compare yoga with stretching practices such as static dynamic, ballistic, and PNF, because stretching is only one component of yoga. Furthermore, there are many types of yoga that may place greater emphasis on holding positions for longer to achieve changes in connective tissue (e.g. yin yoga) or place greater emphasis on breathing patterns or meditation.

Unfortunately, science is messy and the results are not always consistent. The same interventions and measures can be used on sedentary women and men, young people, young adults, and seniors, trained and untrained, and you can get different results in every study. How do you figure out what is right? How do you know what to do? Meta-analyses are usually considered the gold standard for integrating all the disparate information in the literature into a cogent, understandable, main message. But the problem with meta-analyses is that, sometimes, they might hide some intricacies. Maybe for the general population of sedentary and recreationally trained people, static and PNF stretching provide the greatest ROM increases. But as gymnasts, figure skaters, and circus acrobats are the extremes of the population, possibly just for them ballistic stretching is more important because it emulates actions used in their sport. I have used those extreme athletes as a fictional example. There is very little research on such a small population of extreme flexibility athletes. If a meta-analysis looked at 30, 50, or 100 papers and only 2 or 3 dealt with such highly trained athletes, then their responses to specific stretching could be hidden within the greater numbers of the other studies. A good meta-analysis should highlight these outliers but not all reviews accomplish it.

Thus, based on the information provided in the previous paragraph, it would seem that, in general or on average, PNF and static stretching might provide the greatest increases in ROM. However, later we examine how prolonged static and PNF stretching without a full warm-up protocol might impair subsequent performance. Thus, you need to ask yourself whether you need the utmost ROM. If you are jogging, the amplitude of your stride length is limited and there is no need to have an extreme ROM. Hence, some dynamic stretching before the running might be sufficient. If you are resistance training, and for your squat warm-up you take a light weight or just your body mass and go through a full ROM for 10 repetitions, then that might be sufficient because you will not exceed that range while lifting. A study by Morton et al. (88) compared 5 weeks of resistance training to static stretch training and found improved ROM in both groups, with no significant differences between the groups in the flexibility of the hamstrings, hip flexors and extensors, or shoulder extensors. Thus, the ROM with resistance training was sufficient to provide a similar flexibility training adaptation as a stretching programme. Another study incorporated dancers who either resistance trained, or stretched at a low intensity (3/10) or a moderate-to-high intensity (8/10) for 6 weeks (89). All groups improved their passive ROM with no difference between groups, whereas the resistance trained and low-intensity stretch-training groups improved their active ROM. The authors suggested that dance instructors and coaches should incorporate stretching and end-of-range resistance training within their schedules, incorporating stretching at the end of the recovery session. They also recommended that the position of the stretches is very important in order to eliminate muscle contractions, so the body should be in a stable position without extraneous tension. Each stretch, according to this study, should be held for 60 seconds at an intensity of 3/10.

The warm-up is not a time to try to make plastic (semi-permanent) changes in your flexibility. The warm-up prepares you for the upcoming activity. There is no need to be able to do the Russian splits (legs completely abducted until they are horizontal on the floor) before a 5-km jog or step-ups in the weight room. However, if you have back problems because you spend 8 hours per day sitting at a computer, and now your pelvis has an anterior tilt due to shortened hip flexors affecting your lumbar spinal curvature, then the use of static or PNF stretching as a separate flexibility workout might be in order.

Range of motion norms

The average passive joint ROMs have been provided in a few studies. Tables 3.1–3.5 provide a comparison of a sample of these studies in healthy or normal individuals.

Measuring ROM

There are a myriad of instruments that can be used to measure ROM. Most individuals do not have access to advanced scientific laboratories, so the universal, full-circle goniometer is one of the most preferred pieces of equipment for measuring ROM (13) (Figure 3.5). The use of goniometers has been evaluated as having high reliability (intraclass correlation coefficients [ICC]) of >0.91(13). Although instruments can have strong time-to-time (intrarater) reliability they may not have good between-instrument reliability, e.g. a universal, fluid, and electronic goniometer were tested for reliability (90). Although the intertester reliability in Goodwin's study was excellent ($r = 0.90$–0.93), the reliability scores between instruments were not as consistent.

Fluid goniometer vs universal goniometer = 0.90
Fluid goniometer vs electrogoniometer = 0.33
Universal goniometer vs electrogoniometer = 0.51

Another study compared a standard plastic goniometer with a fleximeter (gravitation-based ROM-measuring device) or inclinometer (Figure 3.6). The fleximeter/inclinometer demonstrated moderate-to-excellent intra- and interrater reliability, but the goniometer showed poor-to-moderate intra- and interrater reliability (91). These findings indicate that, if just one device is used to measure differences before and after stretching or training, the extent of change should be reliable but you cannot always interchangeably use these devices to monitor flexibilitydifferences. Similar conclusions were made when comparing goniometers and a digital level

TABLE 3.1 Upper limb and back passive ROM (Family Medical Practice)

Joint	Motion	Family Medical Practice (°)	Heyward (2005) (°)
Shoulder	Flexion	180	150–180
	Extension	45–60	50–60
	Abduction	150	180
	External rotation	90	90
	Internal rotation	70–90	70–90
Elbow	Flexion		140–150
	Extension		0
Radioulnar	Pronation		80
	Supination		80
Wrist	Flexion		60–80
	Extension		60–70
	Radial deviation		20
	Ulnar deviation		30
Cervical spine	Flexion		45–60
	Extension		45–75
	Lateral flexion		45
	Rotation		60–80
Thoracolumbar spine	Flexion		60–80
	Extension		20–30
	Lateral flexion		25–35
	Rotation		30–45

Source: (www.fpnotebook.com/Ortho/Exam/ShldrRngOfMtn.htm)
Heyward VH. *Advanced fitness assessment and exercise prescription.* Windsor, Ontario: Human Kinetics Publishers, 2005.

TABLE 3.2 Lower body passive ROM

Joint	Motion	Roass and Andersson (1982) (°)	American Association of Orthopedic Surgeons (1969) (°)	Boone and Azen (1979) (°)	Heyward (2005) (°)	Hallaceli et al. (2014) (°)
Hip	Extension	9.5	28	12.1	30	19.8
	Flexion	120.4	113	121.3	100–120	128.8
	Abduction	38.8	48	40.5	40–45	45.7
	Adduction	30.5	31	25.6	20–30	24.2
	Internal Rotation	32.6	35	44.4	40–45	43.4
	External Rotation	33.7	48	44.2	45–50	41.9

(*Continued*)

TABLE 3.2 (Cont.)

Joint	Motion	Roass and Andersson (1982) (°)	American Association of Orthopedic Surgeons (1969) (°)	Boone and Azen (1979) (°)	Heyward (2005) (°)	Hallaceli et al. (2014) (°)
Knee	Extension		10		0–10	7.53
	Flexion	143.8	134	141	135–150	142.4
Ankle	Extension (dorsiflexion)	15.3	18	12.2	20	22.5
	Flexion (plantar flexion)	39.7	48	54.3	40–50	49.99
	Valgus (eversion)	27.9	18	19.2	15–20	19.9
	Varus (inversion)	27.8	33	36.2	30–35	34.1

Source: American Academy of Orthopaedic Surgeons. *Joint motion: Method of measuring and recording*, 4th reprint. Edinburgh: E. & S. Livingstone Ltd, 1965.
Boone DC and Azen SP. Normal range of motion of joints in male subjects. *J Bone Joint Surg Am* 61, 756–759, 1979.
Hallaceli H, Uruc V, Uysal HH, Ozden R, Hallaceli C, Soyuer F, et al. Normal hip, knee and ankle range of motion in the Turkish population. *Acta Orthop Traumatol Turc* 48, 37–42, 2014.
Heyward VH. *Advanced Fitness assessment and exercise prescription*. Windsor, Ontario: Human Kinetics Publishers, 2005.
Moller MEJ, Oberg B and Gillquist J. Duration of stretching effect on range of motion in lower extremities. *Arch Phys Med Rehabil*, 3, 171–173, 1985.
Roaas A and Andersson GB. Normal range of motion of the hip, knee and ankle joints in male subjects, 30-40 years of age. *Acta Orthop Scand* 53, 205–208, 1982.

(92). Whereas intratester reliability ranged from 0.91 to 0.99, intertester reliability (ICC) ranged from 0.31 to 0.95, with limits 2.3 times higher for intertester reliability when testing for various shoulder movements (external and internal rotation and flexion). The authors indicated that experienced individuals using the same instrument for repeated measures (goniometer or digital level) should be able to detect a shoulder ROM change of at least 6°, but when comparing measures from two people, the detectable change is 15°. Another study (93) examined the reliability of measuring ROM with visual estimation, goniometry, still photography, "stand and reach," and hand behind back reach for six different shoulder movements. In general, they reported fair-to-good reliability ($r = 0.53–0.73$) for visual estimation, goniometry, still photography, and stand and reach. However, the tests had standard errors of measurement between 14 and 25° (interrater trial) and 11 and 23° (intrarater trial). The hand-behind-the-back test showed poor interrater and intrarater reliability ($r = 0.14–0.39$). These poor findings are probably related to the number of joints involved and the complexity of movement. Not all

TABLE 3.3 Norms for joint range of motion using Leighton fleximeter (Leighton, 1987)

Joint movement	Males					Females				
	Low	Moderately low (°)	Average (°)	Moderately high (°)	High (°)	Low (°)	Moderately low (°)	Average (°)	Moderately high (°)	High (°)
Neck										
Flexion/extension	<107	107–128	129–142	143–160	>160	<125	125–141	142–160	161–177	>177
Lateral flexion	<74	74–89	90–106	107–122	>122	<84	84–99	100–116	117–132	>132
Rotation	<141	141–160	161–181	182–210	>201	<158	158–177	178–198	199–218	>218
Shoulder										
Flexion/extension	<207	207–223	224–242	243–259	>259	<226	226–242	243–261	262–278	>278
Adduction/abduction	<158	158–171	172–186	187–200	>200	<167	167–180	181–195	196–209	>209
Rotation	<154	154–171	172–192	193–210	>210	<189	189–206	207–227	228–245	>245
Elbow										
Flexion/extension	<133	133–143	144–156	157–167	>167	<133	133–143	144–156	157–167	>167
Forearm										
Supination/pronation	<151	151–170	171–191	192–211	>211	<160	160–179	180–200	201–220	>220
Wrist										
Flexion/extension	<112	112–131	132–152	153–172	>172	<136	136–155	156–176	177–196	>196
Ulnar/radial deviation	<64	64–77	78–92	93–105	>105	<75	75–88	89–101	102–117	>117

Hip									
Flexion/Extension	<50	50–67	68–88	89–106	>106	<82	82–99	100–120	121–138	>138
Adduction/abduction	<41	41–50	51–61	62–71	>71	<45	45–54	55–65	66–75	>75
Rotation	<59	59–78	79–99	100–119	>119	<90	90–109	110–130	131–150	>150
Knee									
Flexion/extension	<122	122–133	134–146	147–157	>157	<134	134–144	145–157	158–168	>168
Ankle									
Plantar flexion/dorsiflexion	<48	48–58	59–71	72–82	>82	<56	56–66	67–79	80–90	>90
Inversion/eversion	<30	30–41	42–56	57–68	>68	<39	39–50	51–65	66–77	>77
Trunk									
Flexion/extension	<45	45–62	63–83	84–101	>101	<30	30–47	48–68	69–86	>86
Lateral flexion	<75	74–89	90–106	107–122	>122	<104	104–119	120–136	137–152	>152
Rotation	<108	108–126	127–147	148–166	>166	<134	134–152	153–173	174–192	>192

Source: Leighton B. *Manual of Instruction for the Leighton Flexmeter*. 1987.

TABLE 3.4 Percentile ranks for the sit-and-reach test (Hoffman, 2006)

Percentile rank	Age (years) 20–29		30–39		40–49		50–59		60–69	
	M (cm)	F (cm)	M (cm)	F (cm)	M (cm)	F (cm)	M (cm)	F (cm)	M (cm)	F (cm)
90	39	40	37	39	34	37	35	37	32	34
80	35	37	34	36	31	33	29	34	27	31
70	33	35	31	34	27	32	26	32	23	28
60	30	33	29	32	25	30	24	29	21	27
50	28	31	26	30	22	28	22	27	19	25
40	26	29	24	28	20	26	19	26	15	23
30	23	26	21	25	17	23	15	23	13	21
20	20	23	18	22	13	21	12	20	11	20
10	15	19	14	18	9	16	9	16	8	15

Source: Hoffman J. *Norms for fitness, performance, and health*. Champaign, IL: Human Kinetics, 2006.

TABLE 3.5 Percentile ranks for the modified sit-and-reach test (Hoffman, 2006)

Percentile rank	Females <18 years		19–35 years		36–49 years		>50 years	
	(inches)	(cm)	(inches)	(cm)	(inches)	(cm)	(inches)	(cm)
99	22.6	57.4	21.0	53.3	19.8	50.3	17.2	43.7
95	19.5	49.5	19.3	49.0	19.2	48.8	15.7	39.9
90	18.7	47.5	17.9	45.5	17.4	44.2	15.0	38.1
80	17.8	45.2	16.7	42.4	16.2	41.1	14.2	36.1
70	16.5	41.9	16.2	41.1	15.2	38.6	13.6	34.5
60	16.0	40.6	15.8	40.1	14.5	36.8	12.3	31.2
50	15.2	38.6	14.8	37.6	13.5	34.3	11.1	28.2
40	14.5	36.8	14.5	36.8	12.8	32.5	10.1	25.7
30	13.7	34.8	13.7	34.8	12.2	31.0	9.2	23.4
20	12.6	32.0	12.6	32.0	11.0	27.9	8.3	21.2
10	11.4	29.0	10.1	25.7	9.7	24.6	7.5	19.1
	Males							
99	20.1	51.1	24.7	62.7	18.9	48.0	16.2	41.1
95	19.6	49.8	18.9	48.0	18.2	46.2	15.8	40.1
90	18.2	46.2	17.2	43.7	16.1	40.9	15.0	38.1
80	17.8	45.2	17.0	43.2	14.6	37.1	13.3	33.8
70	16.0	40.6	15.8	40.1	13.9	35.3	12.3	31.2
60	15.2	38.6	15.0	38.1	13.4	34.0	11.5	29.2
50	14.5	36.8	14.4	36.6	12.6	32.0	10.2	25.9

(Continued)

TABLE 3.5 (Cont.)

	Males							
40	14.0	35.6	13.5	34.3	11.6	29.5	9.7	24.6
30	13.4	34.0	13.0	33.0	10.8	27.4	9.3	23.6
20	11.8	30.0	11.6	29.5	9.9	25.1	8.8	22.4
10	9.5	24.1	9.2	23.4	8.3	21.1	7.8	19.8

Source: Hoffman J. *Norms for fitness, performance, and health.* Champaign, IL: Human Kinetics, 2006.

studies recommend visual inspection because van de Pol (94) stated that measurements of physiological ROM using goniometers or inclinometers were more reliable than using vision. However, another review reported that inter-rater reliability of lower-extremity, passive ROM measurement is generally low (95). One of the major problems is the sensation or measurements of end-feel, which is a term used to describe the extent of sensation on the hands of the examiner when they move the passive joint to the supposed end of ROM. Active ROM is reported to have higher reliability than passive ROM because passive measures depend on the force applied to the limbs by another individual, and that force and sensations can change unconsciously between trials and significantly between individuals.

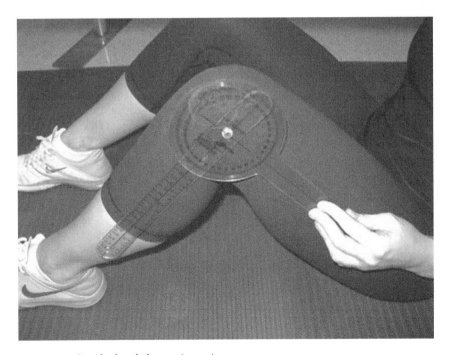

FIGURE 3.5 Standard and electronic goniometers

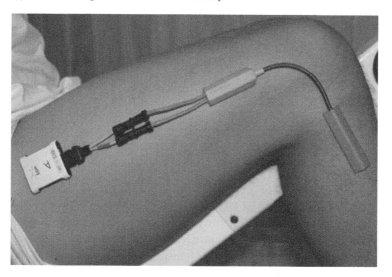

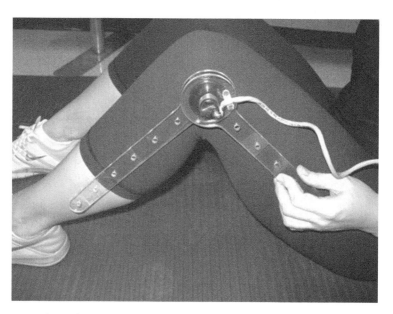

FIGURE 3.5 (Cont.)

Sometimes ROM tests may not measure what most people think they should measure. The ubiquitous sit-and-reach test is commonly used to measure lower back and hamstring flexibility (Figure 3.7). Although a number of studies report that the sit-and-reach test has moderate (96,97) or strong (98) validity for measuring hamstring extensibility, but low validity for lumbar spine extensibility (99), another study contradicts this and states that the sit-and-reach test (as

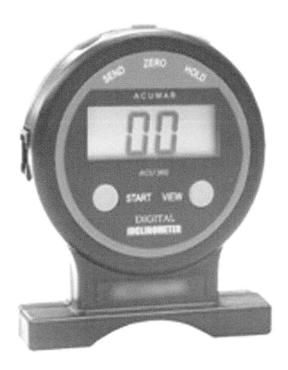

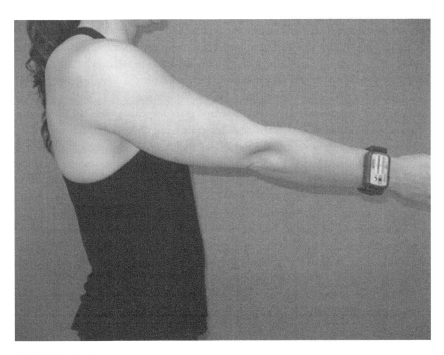

FIGURE 3.6 Inclinometers

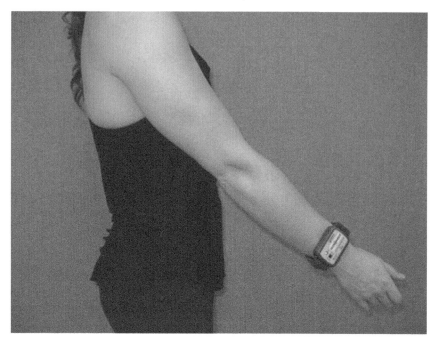

FIGURE 3.6   (Cont.)

well as the toe-touch test) is a more appropriate measure of lumbar spinal flexibility and pelvic-tilt ROM, but not appropriate for hamstring flexibility (100). These results instil confusion into the general population. The sit-and-reach test and toe-touch test can conceivably place undue pressure on the vertebral discs (101), leading to injury. These concerns led to the development of the "back-saver" sit-and-reach test, where only one leg (hamstring) is stretched at a time (102). Another variation is the chair sit-and-reach test (reliability: $r = 0.76$–0.81), for which the individual, while seated on the front edge of the chair, extends one leg with the other leg flexed to the side (103). The individual at the same time reaches as far forward as possible. Furthermore, scapular abduction or arm-length differences could also affect sit-and-reach scores (104). Hence, a "modified" sit-and-reach test (105) was introduced in which the score is based on the difference between the initial starting touch point of the fingers on the device from a straight-back (good posture) seated position and their maximum reach, rather than just the maximum reach, which is commonly measured in the non-modified sit-and-reach tests. Finally, it has also been argued that taller individuals can reach further than shorter individuals with the sit-and-reach test because a longer spine permits greater spinal flexion (106). Obviously, no test is perfectly valid or reliable but, in general, the articles tend to indicate that, if you use one particular test throughout, then it will be fairly reliable at detecting change over time, but it is difficult and precarious to compare the scores between one test and another.

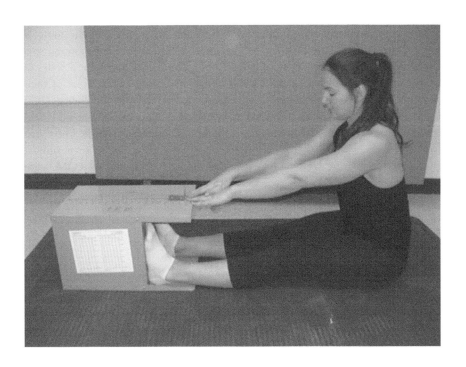

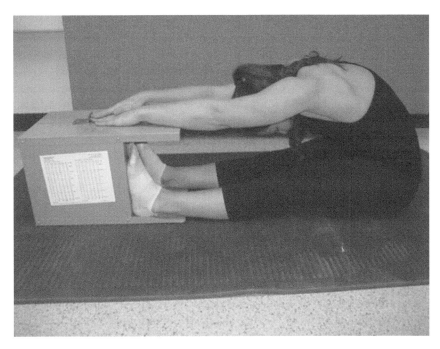

FIGURE 3.7 Sit-and-reach test

It is very important when monitoring flexibility to ensure that the joint or joints to be measured are isolated and that other joints are not contributing to a functional ROM. Individuals who lack flexibility or ROM in one or a series of joints can sometimes compensate by using or emphasizing another part of their body that has better flexibility. This compensatory relative flexibility (107) assumes that the individual will want to move through a movement or ROM with the least resistance. Thus, when measuring hip extensor ROM in a pronated position, if the individual has tight quadriceps, they may extend their lumbar spine to achieve a greater score or, if measuring supine hip flexor ROM, with tight hamstrings they could posteriorly tilt their pelvis to help increase the movement of their leg. When performing an activity, the individual may compensate for their lack of flexibility by relying on another body segment not well designed for the movement and this could lead to injuries (1).

Sex differences

It is common knowledge that most women have better flexibility than the average man (108–113). Some factors contributing to this difference could be differences in muscle mass, joint geometry, and the degree of collagen in the musculotendinous unit (MTU) (1). For instance, men with highly hypertrophied biceps brachii or hamstrings may be restricted by the muscle mass from achieving a full elbow-flexion or knee-flexion ROM. Women show greater hip flexibility with a single leg-raise test (114). The broader and shallower hips of women contribute to this greater flexibility (1). Pelvic and thoracic angles are also greater in women (115). Not all tests ratify these assumptions. For example, in one study, men demonstrated equal sit-and-reach test scores as women but the women had 8% greater pelvic flexion (115). Men tend to possess higher musculotendinous stiffness (116), which would increase the resistance to a higher ROM. One study reported 44% greater gastrocnemius stiffness in men (18). Lower female passive muscle stiffness may be attributed to lesser female muscle cross-sectional area and thickness (117,118) or an intrinsically more compliant female muscle (lower viscoelastic properties) (18). Female tendons have greater compliance than male ones (119). Women are reported to have lower collagen fibril concentrations and percentage area compared with males (120). Collagen is a major component of skin, fascia, cartilage, ligaments, skin, tendons, and bones. It is a protein composed of a triple helix, giving it high tensile strength. The elasticity modulus is highly correlated with fibril concentration (120).

Some studies report an association between the greater tendon compliance of women and their oestrogen secretion (121). Other endocrine differences occur with pregnancy. Women become more flexible during pregnancy due to the release of various hormones such as relaxin, which allows greater extensibility of the interpubic ligament; however, not all studies agree (1). Without this increased flexibility, the relatively large skull of the baby would never make it through the vaginal canal. This relaxin-induced increase in flexibility can also affect the ROM of other joints throughout the body (1).

After an acute bout of passive stretching (135 seconds), women demonstrated greater ROM increases, which were attributed to a greater stretch tolerance because their musculotendinous stiffness did not change with the stretching (116). Generally, in order to obtain similar ROM increases as women, men may need to stretch at a higher intensity or longer duration (116).

Ageing differences

Ageing or senescence has been described as a "process of unfavourable progressive change" (122). Some older adults, as they look in the mirror, might counter that it is a depressive (psychologically and physiologically) rather than a progressive change that alters their previously younger, wrinkle-free skin, decreases their strength, power, and speed, and increases their joint, ligament, and musculotendinous stiffness. Older adults tend to be less flexible than their younger counterparts (48,65). However, when they participate in stretch training programmes, their relative increases in flexibility are similar to young adults (65). Furthermore, trained older adults demonstrate greater degrees of flexibility than untrained older adults (65). As with other physical fitness parameters, the typically more sedentary lifestyle of senior adults exacerbates the decline in flexibility. A lack of activity can affect the synthesis, degradation, and interconnections between connective tissue.

Collagen consists of long, fibrous structural proteins with high tensile strength and is the main component of fascia, cartilage, ligaments, tendons, bone. and skin (123) (Figure 3.8). It is an evolutionary ancient protein involved with the binding of cells of the simplest animals, such as sponges, as well as humans (124). Collagen has an extremely low compliance, similar to the tensile characteristics of copper. Intermolecular cross-links stabilize collagen, preventing the long rod-like

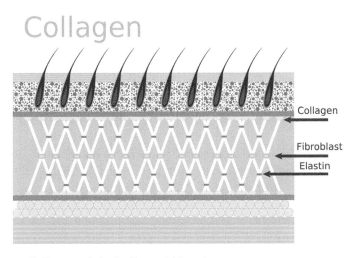

FIGURE 3.8   Collagen and elastin fibres within a tissue

molecules from sliding past each other, forming almost inextensible fibres (125). In combination with the proteins – elastin and soft keratin – their mix provides not only strength (collagen) but also elasticity (elastin) (126). Unlike collagen, elastin can double its length (125). With ageing, collagen increases markedly (126), which would have significant effects on ROM. The low compliance of collagen increases muscle, tendon, and ligament stiffness. Thus, with increased stiffness or lower compliance, higher passive tension occurs for smaller increases in musculotendinous length. These changes would also have significant effects on the stretch-shortening cycle. An increase in connective tissue proteins such as collagen impede the muscle contraction/relaxation process because it would have less extensible and compressible spring-like capabilities (126). A further complication is the excessive formation of intermolecular cross-links (124). Collagen and elastin cross-links in younger people promote strength and elasticity in the tissue, but excessive cross-links with ageing can ensure that stiffness predominates over compliance. Another age-related change is the decreased hydration (water content) of aged tissue. Proteoglycans (i.e. chondroitin sulphate and keratin), which are present in virtually all extracellular matrices of connective tissues, can hold large amounts of water, and so changes in their composition could lead to mild dehydration and some loss of function and extensibility (124). An example of this lack of extensibility with age can be seen with a simple test. Have a young person (especially a child) and a senior adult pinch the skin on the back of the hand. Then, quickly release the skin and be aware of the time it takes for the skin to return to its original shape and position. In a young child, it is practically instantaneous and would be almost impossible to measure with a stop watch or timer. With a senior adult, you can easily see and measure the slow return of the pinched skin to its original position. The older person's more dehydrated, cross-linked, collagen-predominant skin lacks the elasticity of the young person's skin. The same processes occur in the older person's connective tissues subcutaneously (under the skin) with the muscles, tendons, ligaments, and other tissues.

However, as mentioned, this decreased ROM is attenuated in trained and more active older adults and with stretch-training programmes. Coincidentally, animal studies have shown that the soleus muscles of rats do not get stiffer or as stiff with ageing and possess, relatively, the same stiffness as young rat soleus muscles (126). How can this be? Rats in laboratories love to run on their little treadmills. The soleus muscle would be one of their most highly active muscles. Thus, just like active or trained humans, if the muscle activity is maintained throughout life, the degree of musculotendinous degradation and stiffness is decreased. In a typical inactive older adult, the more elastic-like elastin proteins degrade at a faster rate and are replaced by collagen. In senior-age trained individuals, there would be less degradation, more elastin protein synthesis, less collagen replacement, and less unsuitable cross-linkages. In addition, trained older adults have greater stretch tolerance (i.e. greater tolerance of passive joint moment), so they can push themselves farther while tolerating the relative discomfort (127).

Youth differences

It is generally considered that children have better flexibility than adults. However, more age-specific research has shown different patterns with pre-pubescence and pubescence. Younger children around the age of 5 years typically show a high level of flexibility, which declines progressively until the age of 12 years. During puberty until pre-adulthood 12–18 years), their flexibility exhibits improvements (128–131). Even with very young children when comparing 5-year-old children versus 6-year-old children (109) or kindergarten to second grade children (132), there has been evidence of decreases in flexibility. Not all studies provide a consistent picture. In contrast to the early studies that reported improved flexibility throughout puberty, others have reported decrements (133–138) or no significant change (139,140). Similar to senior adults who experience decrements in strength, power, and ROM, many of the impairments can be related to their activity levels. A similar relationship seems to exist with children with the less active experiencing great ROM deficits. Young and pubescent children who partake in extensive flexibility programmes such as gymnasts, dancers, figure skaters, and others can exhibit astounding levels of flexibility, continually improving from young childhood and through puberty. Other less active children may lose their natural flexibility due to the time spent sitting in school and at home (141,142).

It has been suggested that diminished flexibility during puberty, as well as so-called "growth pains" and "tightness," might be attributed to a greater growth rate of the skeletal bones compared with the growth rate of muscles and connective tissue (143–146). However, a number of studies dispute this common belief, citing in one study that older adolescents actually had greater flexibility (147) and a study of 600 13- to 14-year-old students indicated that, although a decrease in flexibility is associated with growth, growth does not reduce flexibility (141). Furthermore, "growth pains" normally occur before the peak height velocity stage and thus have no connection with growth (148). Regardless of the association or lack of association with growth, one study reported that stretching reduced the duration of "growing pains" in 5- to 14-year-old children (149).

Genetic differences

Claude Bouchard, originally from Quebec, Canada, is internationally renowned for his early genetic studies with twins. His review (150) examined the effect of genetics on flexibility. The flexibility relationship in his studies and others were quite low. Whereas two studies from the same researcher reported moderate-to-strong correlations between 11- to 15-year-old male twins (0.69) (151) and 12- to 17-year-old male and female twins for trunk, hip, and shoulder flexibility (0.7–0.91) (151), most other twin studies found weak correlations (0.18–0.43) (152–155). These results again point to the importance of the environment (nature vs nurture), i.e. the activity levels and flexibility training of individuals play a more important role than their genetics in affecting ROM.

Limb dominance differences

A similar activity-related rationale may be attributed to reports of differences in ROM with dominant versus non-dominant limbs. Two tennis studies (10,156) reported decreased internal rotation of the shoulder but increased external rotation ROM of the dominant arm. Two baseball studies reported either no major differences between right and left sides (157) versus greater hip flexion and internal rotation of the stance leg with baseball pitchers (158). There is conflict in the literature, with some studies showing insignificant or small ROM differences with pubescent and young adult females' shoulders and lower extremities (131), and no differences in ankle dorsiflexion and plantar flexion ROM with 15–34 year olds (159). Other studies report lateralized differences with less right wrist mobility and left hip rotation (108), and greater dominant limb humeral head retroversion angle (160). Rather than limb-side differences in ROM being due to a lateralized predisposition, it seems that differences are more likely to be attributed to a specific, unilateral, expanded dynamic ROM (increased ROM) or higher incidence of injury to a predominant limb during repetitive tasks (decreased ROM).

Circadian (diurnal, time of day) differences

Restricted ROM seems to be more prevalent in the morning (161–169). As the individual becomes more active during the day and increases their core temperature, there will be decreases in viscoelasticity (thixotropic effects: see Chapter 4 for more details), increased tissue compliance, and less resistance to motion. Diurnal fluctuations in endocrine responses (i.e. adrenaline, noradrenaline, thyroid hormones, testosterone, insulin-like growth factors, growth hormone) (170) would also impact basal metabolic activity, contributing to core heat flux changes during the day. As the individual becomes less active and the endocrine activity subsides later in the evening in preparation for sleep, flexibility also diminishes (164). In order to maintain a suitable ROM towards evening, an individual would need to maintain or increase activity in an attempt to maintain a higher body temperature and sustain the energy facilitating hormones (i.e. adrenaline, noradrenaline, thyroid hormones, testosterone, insulin-like growth factors, growth hormone, and others).

Summary

Flexibility, defined as the ROM around a joint, can be altered with passive and active static, dynamic, and PNF stretching as well as other techniques. These stretching techniques can provide elastic (acute or non-permanent) or plastic (semi-permanent with prolonged training) changes to joint flexibility. Most studies show that static and PNF stretching provide greater increases in ROM versus dynamic stretching. Yoga is also very effective for improving ROM, although yoga integrates more diverse activities than just stretching (i.e. breathing techniques, static and prolonged static contractions, and meditation, among other activities), which can affect overall relaxation (enhanced parasympathetic stimulation). Normative data for joint ROM are provided in a number of texts and articles. Most measurement techniques such as the use of goniometers, fleximeters, inclinometers, photography, and sit (stand)-and-reach tests display high reliability, but may not provide similar between-device values.

Women tend to have greater joint ROM than men due to anatomical differences, less musculotendinous unit stiffness (greater compliance), and endocrine differences. With ageing, people tend to become less flexible which may be related to increased collagen proportions and protein cross-linkages. However, much of the flexibility impairments can be attributed to greater inactivity. Youths, on the other hand, tend to have higher flexibility levels which may decrease during puberty compared with childhood. Once again, however, the lower levels of flexibility with puberty can be related to more inactivity. With regard to the effect of genetics on flexibility, activity again plays a more important role than DNA because studies have shown weak-to-strong correlations. Individuals tend to be less flexible in the morning because the core temperature is lower and the relatively long period of inactivity tends to restrict movement.

References

1. Alter MJ. *Science of flexibility*. Champaign, IL: Human Kinetics Publishers, 1996.
2. De V, HA. *Physiology of exercise*. Duboque, IA: Wm C. Brown, 1986.
3. Hebbelink M. *Flexibility*. Oxford: Blackwell Scientific, 1988.
4. Hubley-Kozey CL. Testing flexibility. In: *Physiological testing of the high performance athlete*. MacDougall JD, Weger HA, Green HJ, eds. Champaign, IL: Human Kinetics, 1991, pp 309–359.
5. Liemohn WP. Flexibility and muscular strength. *J Phys Educ Recreat Dance* 59: 37–40, 1988.
6. Stone, Kraemer WJ and Kroll WA. *Sports conditioning and weight training: Programs for an athletic competition*. Dubuque, IA: Wm C. Brown, 1991.
7. Saal JS. Flexibility training. In: *Functional rehabilitation of sports and musculoskeletal injuries*. Gaithersburg, MA Aspen, 1998, pp 84–97.
8. Kent M. *The Oxford dictionary of sports science and medicine*. Oxford: Oxford University Press, 1998.
9. Kisner C and Colby LA. *Therapeutic exercise foundations and techniques*. Philadelphia, PA: F.A. Davis, 2002.
10. Chandler TJ, Kibler WB, Uhl TL, Wooten B, Kiser A, and Stone E. Flexibility comparisons of junior elite tennis players to other athletes. *Am J Sports Med* 18: 134–136, 1990.
11. Halvorson GA. Principles of rehabilitating sports injuries. In: *Scientific foundations of sports medicine*. Teitz CC, ed. Philadelphia, PA: Decker, 1989, pp 345–371.
12. Halbertsma J, Bolhuis A, and Goeken L. Sport stretching: Effect of passive muscle stiffness of short hamstrings. *Arch Phys Med Rehabil* 77: 688–692, 1996.

13. Gajdosik RL and Bohannon RW. Clinical measurement of range of motion. Review of goniometry emphasizing reliability and validity. *Phys Ther* 67: 1867–1872, 1987.

14. Gajdosik RL, Vander Linden DW, and Williams AK. Influence of age on length and passive elastic stiffness characteristics of the calf muscle-tendon unit of women. *Phys Ther* 79: 827–838, 1999.

15. Magnusson SP, Aagaard P, and Nielson JJ. Passive energy return after repeated stretches of the hamstring muscle-tendon unit. *Med Sci Sports Exerc* 32: 1160–1164, 2000.

16. Marshall PW, Cashman A, and Cheema BS. A randomized controlled trial for the effect of passive stretching on measures of hamstring extensibility, passive stiffness, strength, and stretch tolerance. *J Sci Med Sport* 14: 535–540, 2011.

17. Mizuno T, Matsumoto M, and Umemura Y. Decrements in stiffness are restored within 10 min. *Int J Sports Med* 34: 484–490, 2013.

18. Morse CI. Gender differences in the passive stiffness of the human gastrocnemius muscle during stretch. *Eur J Appl Physiol* 111: 2149–2154, 2011.

19. Nakamura M, Ikezoe T, Takeno Y, and Ichihashi N. Effects of a 4-week static stretch training program on passive stiffness of human gastrocnemius muscle-tendon unit in vivo. *Eur J Appl Physiol* 112: 2749–27552011.

20. Behm DG, Bambury A, Cahill F, and Power K. Effect of acute static stretching on force, balance, reaction time, and movement time. *Med Sci Sports Exerc* 36: 1397–1402, 2004.

21. Behm DG, Blazevich AJ, Kay AD, and McHugh M. Acute effects of muscle stretching on physical performance, range of motion, and injury incidence in healthy active individuals: A systematic review. *Appl Physiol Nutr Metab* 41: 1–11, 2016.

22. Behm DG and Chaouachi A. A review of the acute effects of static and dynamic stretching on performance. *Eur J Appl Physiol* 111: 2633–2651, 2011.

23. Cronin J, Nash M, and Whatman C. The acute effects of hamstring stretching and vibration on dynamic knee joint range of motion and jump performance. *Phys Ther Sport* 9: 89–96, 2008.

24. Bandy WD, Irion JM, and Briggler M. The effect of time and frequency of static stretching on flexibility of the hamstring muscles. *Phys Ther* 77: 1090–1096, 1997.

25. Bandy WD, Irion JM, and Briggler M. The effect of static stretch and dynamic range of motion training on the flexibility of the hamstring muscles. *J Orthop Sports Phys Ther* 27: 295–300, 1998.

26. Power K, Behm D, Cahill F, Carroll M, and Young W. An acute bout of static stretching: Effects on force and jumping performance. *Med Sci Sports Exerc* 36: 1389–1396, 2004.

27. Young WB. The use of static stretching in warm-up for training and competition. *Int J Sports Physiol Perform* 2: 212–216, 2007.

28. Young WB and Behm DG. Effects of running, static stretching and practice jumps on explosive force production and jumping performance. *J Sports Med Phys Fitness* 43: 21–27, 2003.

29. McHugh MP and Cosgrave CH. To stretch or not to stretch: The role of stretching in injury prevention and performance. *Scand J Med Sci Sports* 20: 169–181, 2010.

30. Safran M, Garrett W, Seaber A, Glisson R, and Ribbeck B. The role of warmup in muscular injury prevention. *Am J Sports Med* 16: 123–129, 1988.

31. Safran M, Seaber A, and Garrett W. Warm-up and muscular injury prevention. An update. *Sports Medicine* 8: 239–249, 1989.

32. Smith C. The warm-up procedure: To stretch or not to stretch. A brief review. *J Orthop Sports Phys Ther* 19: 12–17, 1994.
33. Fletcher IM. The effect of different dynamic stretch velocities on jump performance. *Eur J Appl Physiol* 109: 491–498, 2010.
34. Bacurau RF, Monteiro GA, Ugrinowitsch C, Tricoli V, Cabral LF, and Aoki MS. Acute effect of a ballistic and a static stretching exercise bout on flexibility and maximal strength. *J Strength Condit Res* 23: 304–308, 2009.
35. Nelson AG and Kokkonen J. Acute ballistic muscle stretching inhibits maximal strength performance. *Res Q Exerc Sport* 72: 415–419, 2001.
36. Behm DG and Sale DG. Velocity specificity of resistance training. *Sports Med* 15: 374–388, 1993.
37. Sale D and MacDougall JD. Specificity in strength training: A review for the coach and athlete. *Can J Appl Sports Sci* 6: 87–92, 1981.
38. Bishop D. Warm up II: Performance changes following active warm up and how to structure the warm up. *Sports Med – ADIS Int* 33: 483–498, 2003.
39. Fletcher IM and Jones B. The effect of different warm-up stretch protocols on 20 meter sprint performance in trained rugby union players. *J Strength Condit Res* 18: 885–888, 2004.
40. Young W and Behm D. Should static stretching be used during a warm-up for strength and power activities? *Strength Condit J* 24: 33–37, 2002.
41. Guissard N and Duchateau J. Effect of static stretch training on neural and mechanical properties of the human plantar-flexor muscles. *Muscle Nerve* 29: 248–255, 2004.
42. Guissard N and Duchateau J. Neural aspects of muscle stretching. *Exerc Sport Sci Rev* 34: 154–158, 2006.
43. Guissard N, Duchateau J, and Hainaut K. Muscle stretching and motoneuron excitability. *Eur J Appl Physiol* 58: 47–52, 1988.
44. Sherrington CS. Flexion-reflex of the limb, crossed extension reflex stepping and standing. *J Physiol* 40: 28–121, 1910.
45. Sherrington CS. Remarks on some aspects of reflex inhibition. *Proc Royal Soc Lond* 97: 519–519, 1925.
46. Sady SP, Wortman M, and Blanke D. Flexibility training: Ballistic, static or proprioceptive neuromuscular facilitation? *Arch Phys Med Rehabil* 63: 261–263, 1982.
47. Sharman MJ, Cresswell AG, and Riek S. Proprioceptive neuromuscular facilitation stretching: Mechanisms and clinical implications. *Sports Med* 36: 929–939, 2006.
48. Gonzalez-Rave JM, Sanchez-Gomez A, and Santos-Garcia DJ. Efficacy of two different stretch training programs (passive vs. proprioceptive neuromuscular facilitation) on shoulder and hip range of motion in older people. *J Strength Cond Res* 26: 1045–1051, 2012.
49. Hindle KB, Whitcomb TJ, Briggs WO, and Hong J. Proprioceptive neuromuscular facilitation (PNF): Its mechanisms and effects on range of motion and muscular function. *J Hum Kinet* 31: 105–113, 2012.
50. Osternig L, Robertson R, Troxel R, and Hansen P. Differential responses to proprioceptive neuromuscular facilitation (PNF) stretch techniques. *Med Sci Sports Exerc* 22: 106–111, 1990.
51. Thomas E, Bianco A, Paoli A, and Palma A. The relation between stretching typology and stretching duration: The effects on range of motion. *Int J Sports Med* 39: 243–254, 2018.

52. American College of Sports Medicine. ACSM's guidelines for exercise testing and prescription. *Med Sci Sports Exerc* 6: 158–164, 2000.
53. Radford JA, Burns J, Buchbinder R, Landorf KB, and Cook C. Does stretching increase ankle dorsiflexion range of motion? A systematic review. *Br J Sports Med* 40: 870–875, discussion 875, 2006.
54. Magnusson MP. M. H. body height changes with hyperextention. *Clin Biomech* 4: 236–238, 1996.
55. Whatman C, Knappstein A, and Hume P. Acute changes in passive stiffness and range of motion post-stretching. *Phys Ther Sport* 7: 195–200, 2006.
56. Behm DG, Button DC, and Butt JC. Factors affecting force loss with prolonged stretching. *Can J Appl Physiol* 26: 261–272, 2001.
57. Behm DG, Plewe S, Grage P, Rabbani A, Beigi HT, Byrne JM, and Button DC. Relative static stretch-induced impairments and dynamic stretch-induced enhancements are similar in young and middle-aged men. *Appl Physiol Nutr Metab* 36: 790–797, 2011.
58. Fowles JR, Sale DG, and MacDougall JD. Reduced strength after passive stretch of the human plantar flexors. *J Appl Physiol* 89: 1179–1188, 2000.
59. Knudson D. Stretching during warm-up: Do we have enough evidence? *JOPERD* 70: 24–28, 1999.
60. Moller ME, Oberg B, and Gillquist J. Duration of stretching effect on range of motion in lower extremities. *Arch Phys Med Rehabil* 3: 171–173, 1985.
61. Zito M, Driver D, Parker C, and Bohannon R. Lasting effects of one bout of two 15-second passive stretches on ankle dorsiflexion range of motion. *J Orthop Sports Phys Ther* 26: 214–221, 1997.
62. Depino GM, Webright WG, and Arnold BL. Duration of maintained hamstring flexibility after cessation of an acute static stretching protocol. *J Athl Train* 35: 56–59, 2000.
63. Spernoga SG, Uhl TL, Arnold BL, and Gansneder BM. Duration of maintained hamstring flexibility after a one-time, modified hold-relax stretching protocol. *J Athl Train* 36: 44–48, 2001.
64. Etnyre BR and Lee EJ. Chronic and acute flexibility of men and women using 3 different stretching techniques. *Res Q Exerc Sport*, 59: 222–228, 1988.
65. Ferber R, Osternig L, and Gravelle D. Effect of PNF stretch techniques on knee flexor muscle EMG activity in older adults. *J Electromyogr Kinesiol* 12: 391–397, 2002.
66. O'Hora J, Cartwright A, Wade CD, Hough AD, and Shum GL. Efficacy of static stretching and proprioceptive neuromuscular facilitation stretch on hamstrings length after a single session. *J Strength Condit Res/Natl Strength Condit Assoc* 25: 1586–1591, 2011.
67. Condon SM and Hutton RS. Soleus muscle electromyographic activity and ankle dorsi-flexion range of motion during four stretching procedures. *Phys Ther* 67: 24–30, 1987.
68. Maddigan ME, Peach AA, and Behm DG. A comparison of assisted and unassisted proprioceptive neuromuscular facilitation techniques and static stretching. *J Strength Condit Res/Natl Strength Condit Assoc* 26: 1238–1244, 2012.
69. Yuktasir B and Kaya F. Investigation into the long term effects of static and PNF stretching exercises on range of motion and jump preformance. *J Bodywork Movement Ther* 13: 11–21, 2009.
70. Medeiros DM. Comparison between static stretching and proprioceptive neuro-muscular facilitation on hamstring flexibility: Systematic review and meta-analysis. *Eur J Physiother* July 2018.

71. Beedle BB and Mann CL. A comparison of two warm-ups on joint range of motion. *J Strength Cond Res* 21: 776–779, 2007.

72. Perrier ET, Pavol MJ, and Hoffman MA. The acute effects of a warm-up including static or dynamic stretching on countermovement jump height, reaction time, and flexibility. *J Strength Condit Res/Natl Strength Condit Assoc* 25: 1925–1931, 2011.

73. Amiri-Khorasani M, Abu Osman NA, and Yusof A. Acute effect of static and dynamic stretching on hip dynamic range of motion during instep kicking in professional soccer players. *J Strength and Condit Res/Natl Strength Condit Assoc* 25: 1647–1652, 2011.

74. Duncan MJ and Woodfield LA. Acute effects of warm-up protocol on flexibility and vertical jump in children. *J Exerc Physiol* 9: 9–16, 2006.

75. Barroso R, Tricoli V, Santos Gil SD, Ugrinowitsch C, and Roschel H. Maximal strength, number of repetitions, and total volume are differently affected by static-, ballistic-, and proprioceptive neuromuscular facilitation stretching. *J Strength Cond Res* 26: 2432–2437, 2012.

76. Paradisis GP, Pappas PT, Theodorou AS, Zacharogiannis EG, Skordilis EK, and Smirniotou AS. Effects of static and dynamic stretching on sprint and jump performance in boys and girls. *J Strength Condit Res* 28: 154–160, 2014.

77. Samuel MN, Holcomb WR, Guadagnoli MA, Rubley MD, and Wallmann H. Acute effects of static and ballistic stretching on measures of strength and power. *J Strength Cond Res* 22: 1422–1428, 2008.

78. Sekir U, Arabaci R, Akova B, and Kadagan SM. Acute effects of static and dynamic stretching on leg flexor and extensor isokinetic strength in elite women athletes. *Scand J Med Sci Sports* 20: 268–281, 2010.

79. Covert CA, Alexander MP, Petronis JJ, and Davis DS. Comparison of ballistic and static stretching on hamstring muscle length using an equal stretching dose. *J Strength Cond Res* 24: 3008–3014, 2010.

80. Konrad A, Stafilidis S, and Tilp M. Effects of acute static, ballistic, and PNF stretching exercise on the muscle and tendon tissue properties. *Scand J Med Sci Sports* 27: 1070–1080, 2017.

81. Wallin D, Ekblom B, Grahn R, and Nordenberg T. Improvement of muscle flexibility: A comparison between two techniques. *Am J Sports Med* 13: 263–267, 1985.

82. Fasen JM, O'Connor AM, Schwartz SL, Watson JO, Plastaras CT, Garvan CW, Bulcao C, Johnson SC, and Akuthota V. A randomized controlled trial of hamstring stretching: Comparison of four techniques. *J Strength Cond Res* 23: 660–667, 2009.

83. Jensen AM, Ramasamy A, and Hall MW. Improving general flexibility with a mind–body approach: A randomized, controlled trial using neuro emotional technique(R). *J Strength Cond Res* 26: 2103–2112, 2012.

84. Polsgrove MJ, Eggleston BM, and Lockyer RJ. Impact of 10-weeks of yoga practice on flexibility and balance of college athletes. *Int J Yoga* 9: 27–34, 2016.

85. Madanmohan, TDP, Balakumar B, Nambinarayanan TK, Thakur S, Krishnamurthy N, and Chandrabose A. Effect of yoga training on reaction time, respiratory endurance and muscle strength. *Indian J Physiol Pharmacol* 36: 229–233, 1992.

86. Tran MD, Holly RG, Lashbrook J, and Amsterdam EA. Effects of hatha yoga practice on the health-related aspects of physical fitness. *Prev Cardiol* 4: 165–170, 2001.

87. Balaji PA, Varne SR, and Ali SS. Physiological effects of yogic practices and transcendental meditation in health and disease. *N Am J Med Sci* 4: 442–448, 2012.

88. Morton SK, Whitehead JR, Brinkert RH, and Caine DJ. Resistance training vs. static stretching: Effects on flexibility and strength. *J Strength Cond Res* 25: 3391–3398, 2011.

89. Wyon MA, Smith A, and Koutedakis Y. A comparison of strength and stretch interventions on active and passive ranges of movement in dancers: A randomized controlled trial. *J Strength Cond Res* 27: 3053–3059, 2013.
90. Goodwin J, Clark C, Deakes J, Burdon D, and Lawrence C. Clinical methods of goniometry: A comparative study. *Disabil Rehabil* 14: 10–15, 1992.
91. Chaves Tcn HM, Belli, JFC, De Hannai, MCT, Bevilacqua-Grossi D, and De Oleivera, OS. Reliability of fleximetry and goniometry for assessing cervical range of motion among children. *Rev Brazilian Fisioterapa* 12: 183–190, 2008.
92. Mullaney MJ, McHugh MP, Johnson CP, and Tyler TF. Reliability of shoulder range of motion comparing a goniometer to a digital level. *Physiother Theory Pract* 26: 327–333, 2010.
93. Hayes K, Walton JR, Szomor ZR, and Murrell GA. Reliability of five methods for assessing shoulder range of motion. *Aust J Physiother* 47: 289–294, 2001.
94. Van De Pol RJ, Van Trijffel E, and Lucas C. Inter-rater reliability for measurement of passive physiological range of motion of upper extremity joints is better if instruments are used: A systematic review. *J Physiother* 56: 7–17, 2010.
95. Van Trijffel E, Van De Pol RJ, Oostendorp RA, and Lucas C. Inter-rater reliability for measurement of passive physiological movements in lower extremity joints is generally low: A systematic review. *J Physiother* 56: 223–235, 2010.
96. Jackson AW and Baker Aa. The realtionship of the sit and reach test to criterion measures of hamstring and back flexibility in young females. *Res Q Exerc Sport* 3: 183–186, 1986.
97. Mayorga-Vega D, Merino-Marban R, and Viciana J. Criterion-related validity of sit-and-reach tests for estimating hamstring and lumbar extensibility: A meta-analysis. *J Sports Sci Med* 13: 1–14, 2014.
98. Jackson A and Langford NJ. The criterion-related validity of the sit and reach test: Replication and extension of previous findings. *Res Q Exerc Sport* 60: 384–387, 1989.
99. Liemohn WP, Sharpe GL, and Wasserman JF. Lumbosacral movement in the sit-and-reach and in Cailliet's protective-hamstring stretch. *Spine (Phila Pa 1976)* 19: 2127–2130, 1994.
100. Muyor JM, Vaquero-Cristobal R, Alacid F, and Lopez-Minarro PA. Criterion-related validity of sit-and-reach and toe-touch tests as a measure of hamstring extensibility in athletes. *J Strength Cond Res* 28: 546–555, 2014.
101. Cailliet R. *Low back pain syndrome*. Philadelphia, PA: F. A. Davis, 1988.
102. Patterson P, Wiksten DL, Ray L, Flanders C, and Sanphy D. The validity and reliability of the back saver sit-and-reach test in middle school girls and boys. *Res Q Exerc Sport* 67: 448–451, 1996.
103. Jones CJ, Rikli RE, Max J, and Noffal G. The reliability and validity of a chair sit-and-reach test as a measure of hamstring flexibility in older adults. *Res Q Exerc Sport* 69: 338–343, 1998.
104. Hopkins DR. The relationship between selected anthropometric measures and sit-and-reach performance. In: Dance National Measurement Symposium, Houston, TX, 1981.
105. Hopkins DR and Hoeger WWK. The modified sit and reach test. In: *Lifetime physical fitness and wellness: A personalized program*, Englewood, CO: Morton, 1986, pp 47–48.
106. Gatton ML and Pearcy MJ. Kinematics and movement sequencing during flexion of the lumbar spine. *Clin Biomech (Bristol, Avon)* 14: 376–383, 1999.
107. Sahrmann SA. *Diagnosis and treatment of movement impairment syndromes*. St. Louis, USA: Mosby Publishers, 2002.

108. Allander E, Bjornsson OJ, Olafsson O, Sigfusson N, and Thorsteinsson J. Normal range of joint movements in shoulder, hip, wrist and thumb with special reference to side: A comparison between two populations. *Int J Epidemiol* 3: 253–261, 1974.

109. Gabbard C and Tandy R. Body composition and flexibilty amoung prepubescent males and females. *J Hum Mov Stud* 4: 153–159, 1988.

110. Haley SM, Tada WL, and Carmichael EM. Spinal mobility in young children. A normative study. *Phys Ther* 66: 1697–1703, 1986.

111. Jones MA, Buis JM, and Harris ID. Relationship of race and sex to physical and motor measures. *Precept Mot Skills* 1: 169–170, 1986.

112. Soucie JM, Wang C, Forsyth A, Funk S, Denny M, Roach KE, Boone D, and Hemophilia Treatment Center Network. Range of motion measurements: Reference values and a database for comparison studies. *Haemophilia* 17: 500–507, 2011.

113. Youdas JW, Krause DA, Hollman JH, Harmsen WS, and Laskowski E. The influence of gender and age on hamstring muscle length in healthy adults. *J Orthop Sports Phys Ther* 35: 246–252, 2005.

114. Mier CM and Shapiro BS. Sex differences in pelvic and hip flexibility in men and women matched for sit-and-reach score. *J Strength Cond Res* 27: 1031–1035, 2013.

115. Lopez-Minarro PA, Andujar PS, and Rodrnguez-Garcna PL. A comparison of the sit-and-reach test and the back-saver sit-and-reach test in university students. *J Sports Sci Med* 8: 116–122, 2009.

116. Hoge KM, Ryan ED, Costa PB, Herda TJ, Walter AA, Stout JR, and Cramer JT. Gender differences in musculotendinous stiffness and range of motion after an acute bout of stretching. *J Strength Cond Res* 24: 2618–2626, 2010.

117. Kubo K, Kanehisa H, Ito M, and Fukunaga T. Effects of isometric training on the elasticity of human tendon structures in vivo. *J Appl Physiol (1985)* 91: 26–32, 2001.

118. Magnusson SP, Simonsen EB, Aagaard P, Boesen J, Johannsen F, and Kjaer M. Determinants of musculoskeletal flexibility: Viscoelastic properties, cross-sectional area, EMG and stretch tolerance. *Scand J Med Sci Sports* 7: 195–202, 1997.

119. Kubo K, Kanehisa H, and Fukunaga T. Gender differences in the viscoelastic properties of tendon structures. *Eur J Appl Physiol Occup Physiol* 88: 520–526, 2003.

120. Hashemi J, Chandrashekar N, Mansouri H, Slauterbeck JR, and Hardy DM. The human anterior cruciate ligament: Sex differences in ultrastructure and correlation with biomechanical properties. *J Orthop Res* 26: 945–950, 2008.

121. Bryant AL, Clark RA, Bartold S, Murphy A, Bennell KL, Hohmann E, Marshall-Gradisnik S, Payne C, and Crossley KM. Effects of estrogen on the mechanical behavior of the human Achilles tendon in vivo. *J Appl Physiol (1985)* 105: 1035–1043, 2008.

122. Lansing AI. Some physiological aspects of ageing. *Physiol Rev* 31: 274–278, 1978.

123. Buehler MJ. Nature designs tough collagen: Explaining the nanostructure of collagen fibrils. *Proc Natl Acad Sci USA*, 103: 12285–12290, 2006.

124. Bailey AJ. Molecular mechanisms of ageing in connective tissues. *Mech Ageing Dev* 122: 735–755, 2001.

125. Bailey AJ, Light ND, and Atkins ED. Chemical cross-linking restrictions on models for the molecular organization of the collagen fibre. *Nature* 288: 408–410, 1980.

126. Alnaqeeb MA, Al Zaid NS, and Goldspink G. Connective tissue changes and physical properties of developing and ageing skeletal muscle. *J Anat* 139 (Pt 4): 677–689, 1984.

127. Blazevich AJ, Cannavan D, Waugh CM, Fath F, Miller SC, and Kay AD. Neuromuscular factors influencing the maximum stretch limit of the human plantar flexors. *J Appl Physiol* 113: 1446–1455, 2012.

128. Buxton D. Extension of the Kraus-Weber test. *Res Q* 3: 210–217, 1957.

129. Gurewitsch AD and O'Neill MA Flexibility of healthy children. *Arch Phys Ther* 4: 216–221, 1994.

130. Kendall HO and Kendall FP. Normal flexibility according to age groups. *J Bone Joint Surg Am* 30A: 690–694, 1948.

131. Koslow RE. Bilateral flexibility in the upper and lower extremities. *J Hum Mov Stud* 9: 467–472, 1987.

132. Milne C, Seefeldt V, and Reuschlein P. Relationship between grade, sex, race, and motor performance in young children. *Res Q* 47: 726–730, 1976.

133. Clarke HH. Joint and body range of movement. *Phys Fit Res Digest* 5: 16–18, 1975.

134. Docherty D and Bell RD. The relationship between flexibility and linearity measures in boys and girls 6-15 years of age. *J Hum Mov Stud* 11: 279–288, 1985.

135. Germain NW and Blair SN. Variability of shoulder flexion with age, activity and sex. *Am Correct Ther J* 37: 156–160, 1983.

136. Krahenbuhl GS and Martin SL. Adolescent body size and flexibility. *Res Q* 48: 797–799, 1977.

137. Moran HM, Hall MA, Barr A, and Ansell BM. Spinal mobility in the adolescent. *Rheumatol Rehabil* 18: 181–185, 1979.

138. Salminen JJ. The adolescent back. A field survey of 370 finnish schoolchildren. *Acta Paediatr Scand Suppl* 315: 1–122, 1984.

139. Burley LR, Dobell HC, and Farrel BJ. Relations of power, speed, flexibility, and certain anthropometric measures of junior high school girls. *Res Q* 32: 442–448, 1961.

140. Mellin G and Poussa M. Spinal mobility and posture in 8- to 16-year-old children. *J Orthop Res* 10: 211–216, 1992.

141. Feldman D, Shrier I, Rossignol M, and Abenhaim L. Adolescent growth is not associated with changes in flexibility. *Clin J Sport Med* 9: 24–29, 1999.

142. Milne RA and Mireau DR. Hmastrings distensibility in the general population: Relationship to pelvic and low back stresses. *J Manipulative Physiol Ther* 2: 146–150, 1979.

143. Bachrach RM. Injuries to dancer's spine. In: *Dance medicine*. Ryan AJS and Stephens RE, eds. Chicago: Pluribus Press, 1987, pp 243–266.

144. Howse AJG. The young ballet dancer. In: *Dance medicine: A comprehensive guide*. Ryan AJS and Stephens RE, eds. Chicago, IL: Pluribus Press, 1987, pp 107–114.

145. Leard JS. Flexibility and conditioning in the young athlete. In: *Pediatric and adolescent sport medicine*. Micheli LJ, ed. Boston, MA: Little, Brown, 1984, pp 194–210.

146. Micheli LJ. Overuse injuries in children's sports: The growth factor. *Orthop Clin North Am* 14: 337–360, 1983.

147. Pratt M. Strength, flexibility, and maturity in adolescent athletes. *Am J Dis Child* 143: 560–563, 1989.

148. Naish JM and Apley J. "Growing pains": A clinical study of non-arthritic limb pains in children. *Arch Dis Child* 26: 134–140, 1951.

149. Baxter MP and Dulberg C. "Growing pains" in childhood: A proposed treatment. *J Pediatr Orthop* 4: 402–406, 1988.

150. Bouchard C, Malina R, and Pérusse L. *Genetics of fitness and physical performance.* Champaign, IL: Human Kinetics, 1997.

151. Kovar R. *Human variation in motor abilities and genetic analysis.* Prague: Charles University, 1981.

152. Chatterjee S and Das N. Physical and motor fitness in twins. *Jpn J Physiol* 45: 519–534, 1995.

153. Devor EJ and Crawford MH. Family resemblance for neuromuscular performance in a Kansas Mennonite community. *Am J Phys Anthropol* 64: 289–296, 1984.

154. Perusse L, Leblanc C, and Bouchard C. Familial resemblance in lifestyle components: Results from the Canada fitness survey. *Can J Public Health* 79: 201–205, 1988.

155. Perusse L, Leblanc C, and Bouchard C. Inter-generation transmission of physical fitness in the Canadian population. *Can J Sport Sci* 13: 8–14, 1988.

156. Chinn CJ, Priest JD, and Kent BE. Upper extremity range of motion, grip strength, and girth in highly skilled tennis players. *Phys Ther* 54: 474–483, 1974.

157. Gurry M, Pappas A, Michaels J, Maher P, Shakman A, Goldberg R, and Rippe J. A comprehensive preseason fitness evaluation for professional baseball players. *Phys Sportsmed* 13: 63–74, 1985.

158. Tippett SR. Lower extremity strength and active range of motion in college baseball pitchers: A comparison between stance leg and kick leg. *J Orthop Sports Phys Ther* 8: 10–14, 1986.

159. Moseley AM, Crosbie J, and Adams R. Normative data for passive ankle plantarflexion – Dorsiflexion flexibility. *Clin Biomech (Bristol, Avon)* 16: 514–521, 2001.

160. Kronberg M, Brostrom LA, and Soderlund V. Retroversion of the humeral head in the normal shoulder and its relationship to the normal range of motion. *Clin Orthop Relat Res* 253: 113–117, 1990.

161. Baxter C and Reilly T. Influence of time of day on all-out swimming. *Br J Sports Med* 17: 122–127, 1983.

162. Bompa T. *Theory and methodology of training.* Dubuque, IA: Kendall/Hunt, 1990.

163. Dick FW. *Sports training principles.* London: Lepus Bokks. 1980.

164. Gifford LS. Circadian variation in human flexibility and grip strength. *Aust J Physiother* 33: 3–9, 1987.

165. O'Driscoll SL and Tomenson J. The cervical spine. *Clin Rheum Dis* 8: 617–630, 1982.

166. Osolin NG. *Das Training des Leichtathleten.* Berlin: Sportverlag, 1952.

167. Osolin NG. *Sovremennaia systema sportnnoi trenirovky [Athlete's training system for competitions].* Moscow: Phyzkultura i sport, 1971.

168. Russell B, Dix DJ, Haller DL, and Jacobs-El J. Repair of injured skeletal muscle: A molecular approach. *Med Sci Sports Exerc* 24: 189–196, 1992.

169. Wing P, Tsang I, Gagnon F, Susak L, and Gagnon R. Diurnal changes in the profile shape and range of motion of the back. *Spine (Phila Pa 1976)* 17: 761–766, 1992.

170. Kraemer WJ, Ratamess NA, and Nindl BC. Recovery responses of testosterone, growth hormone, and IGF-1 after resistance exercise. *J Appl Physiol* 122: 549–558, 2017.

4

MECHANISMS UNDERLYING ACUTE CHANGES IN RANGE OF MOTION

Thixotropic effects

It is not even necessary to stretch in order to temporarily increase range of motion (ROM). Warming the muscles and tendons will easily improve your elastic flexibility. Even more effective is the inclusion of an aerobic activity or warm-up muscle contractions. The traditional warm-up is typically initiated with a submaximal aerobic component (e.g. running, cycling) to raise the body temperature 1–2°C (1,2). Any study that measures joint ROM before and after almost any activity involving some persistent muscle contractions will detect an increase in ROM. S. Peter Magnusson, a well-respected stretch researcher from Denmark, indicated that the acute effects of stretching in the holding phase of a stretch are due to changes in tissue viscoelasticity. The underlying mechanism for this viscoelastic effect is thixotropy, which occurs when viscous (thicker) fluids become less viscous or more fluid like when agitated, sheared, or stressed. When the stress is removed or desists, then the fluid takes a certain period to return to its original viscous state. Muscle contractions are not very efficient. Only 40–60% of the energy consumed during a contraction contributes to producing force (i.e. myofilament, Ca^{2+}, and Na^+/K^+ pump kinetics), whereas 40–60% is released as heat (3). The muscle contraction-induced increase in temperature of the soft tissues can decrease the viscosity of intracellular and extracellular fluid, providing less resistance to movement. Increases in muscle temperature can occur with higher environmental temperatures, and muscle contractions associated with dynamic stretching movements, isometric contractions during proprioceptive neuromuscular facilitation (PNF) stretching, and to a lesser extent the reflexive contractions of static stretching. Thixotropic effects on viscosity are not just muscle related but, as tendons consist of 55–70% water (4), will also be affected by viscosity changes.

A great analogy for those individuals who live in northern climates is the viscosity of the oil in the car or truck engine when it is extremely cold. If you imagine that the pistons are myosin molecules, both have to move in order to create movement. Oil in very cold temperatures would act more like viscous molasses, providing high resistance to movement of the pistons. A cold muscle would have more viscous sarcoplasm providing higher resistance to the intramuscular proteins such as myosin, titin, and others. The extracellular fluid would also be more viscous when cold and thus provide more resistance to the movement or sliding of muscle fibres, tendons, and fascia. If a car is cold and will not start, you plug in the block heater, which can warm up the oil (decrease viscosity) so the pistons can move. If your muscles are cold, muscle contractions can increase musculotendinous temperatures, decreasing viscosity and resistance to movement. In fact, I have had lazy friends who rather than stretch and actively warm up before a squash game would sit in the sauna to warm their bodies and thus "limber up" (i.e. decrease their musculotendinous and myo-fascial resistance to movement). Athletes playing in cold environments must keep this concept in mind. The colder they become, the less pliability and flexibility will result. Often, you may see or hear an athlete who will disdain from standing by a heater or using a blanket or jacket while on the sidelines in a cold or freezing environment. Their intended approach or message is that they are so psychologically "tough"; they do not need to use the same devices as some "soft" or psychologically "weaker" opponents. As a scientist and a coach, I would rather my athletes stay warm and be psychologically "smart" and physiologically "efficient" because hypothermia (cold) affects not only resistance to movement (flexibility), but also strength, power, rate of force development, endurance, metabolism, and other vital processes for success in the event or sport (5,6).

There are a number of other explanations for the increased ROM immediately after stretching. Depending on whether the stretching is static, PNF, or dynamic, there may be various emphases on whether it is thixotropic, neural, mechanical, or psychological (stretch tolerance).

Neural mechanisms of acute static stretching

According to Nathalie Guissard and Jacques Duchateau (7), two internationally distinguished neuromuscular physiologists from Belgium, the amount of stretch or joint ROM that can be produced is highly attributable to the extent of muscle resistance caused by tonic reflexes. Whereas dynamic movements (not through a full ROM) and dynamic stretching (a full or almost full ROM) tend to excite the neuromuscular system, static stretching is purported to decrease or disfacilitate this reflexive activity excitation of the motoneurons (8–11). The origin of this reflex suppression can be tested by using the Hoffmann reflex (H-reflex) and the tendon reflex (T-reflex) (Figure 4.1). The H-reflex is evoked by stimulation of the Ia fibres to monitor the afferent excitability of the α-motoneurons (12). Decreases in the H-reflex amplitude can signal decreases in motoneuron excitability or presynaptic inhibition (inhibition of interneuron(s) innervating Ia terminals) of the Ia afferents.

Hoffman (H)-reflex and tendon reflex

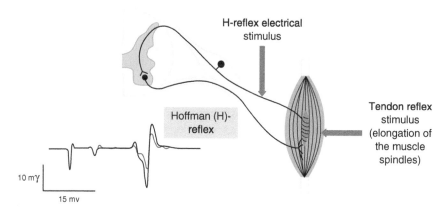

FIGURE 4.1   Hoffman reflex and tendon reflex

What is the difference between inhibition and disfacilitation? Inhibition is a more active process caused by the activation of inhibitory interneurons, leading to inhibitory postsynaptic potentials (IPSPs) in the motoneurons (13). These interneurons would release inhibitory neurotransmitters such as γ-aminobutyric acid (GABA). On the other hand, with disfacilitation, motoneurons would be hyperpolarized due to the temporal absence of excitatory synaptic activity (13). In simpler terms, if you were riding a bicycle and you slowed your pedalling rate or stopped rotating the crank, you would decrease the activity and the speed of the bicycle would be disfacilitated. However, if you applied the brake pads to the wheels, then you would actively attempt to slow the bike, just like an interneuron, and thus you would be inhibiting the bike's speed. The T-reflex could be a combination of inhibition or disfacilitation. It is elicited by tapping (percussion) of the tendon and could be affected by central changes (disfacilitation of motoneuron excitability and presynaptic inhibition) and by changes in the muscle spindle sensitivity/activity (disfacilitation). One hour of repeated passive stretching of the plantar flexors has been shown to decrease the stretch reflex by 85% whereas the H-reflex was reduced by 44% (14). However, you would have to ask, who would ever stretch their calf muscles for an hour. A good example is how lab research that tries to understand mechanisms does not always parallel real life.

With passive static stretching, the muscle is typically extended at a slow-to-moderate rate into an elongated position by another person or device (i.e. rubber band or machine; see Figure 3.1 in Chapter 3). This extended or elongated position is then held for an extended period of time, typically from 15 seconds to 60 seconds (9,15). It is the responsibility of the muscle spindles to detect, continuously monitor, and send signals to the central nervous system about the rate and extent of the muscle elongation (16,17). It can be regarded as both a protective system and a proprioceptive (position sense) system. As a protective system, if the muscle is elongated at a rapid rate to the end or near the end of the ROM, then a reflexive signal will be sent to the spinal cord to contract the muscle that is being stretched (myotactic reflex: Figure 4.2) (18). This reflex is the action of the quadriceps muscle which you experience when a doctor taps your patellar tendon (front of the knee) and then your lower leg jerks forwards (T-reflex). The doctor's hammer has elongated the patellar tendon, which is attached to quadriceps, stretching that muscle, detected by the muscle spindles, and leading to a reflex to the spinal cord which in turn causes your quadriceps to contract. This reflex contraction of the elongated muscle should therefore help prevent the joint skeletal structures (bones and cartilage) and ligaments from exceeding the joint and muscle's functional ROM, and thus help to prevent damage or injury. While the elongated muscle is being reflexively contracted, the antagonist to that muscle is being inhibited. The myotactic reflex is monosynaptic (one synapse), whereas the antagonist inhibition is disynaptic (two synapses). In terms of movement, this antagonist inhibition is efficient because it automatically reduces muscle contractions that work in opposition to the intended motion. Thus, if you are walking, the dynamic contraction and elongation of quadriceps will lead to further excitation of quadriceps, which propels you along while the hamstrings are being inhibited

The Stretch Reflex

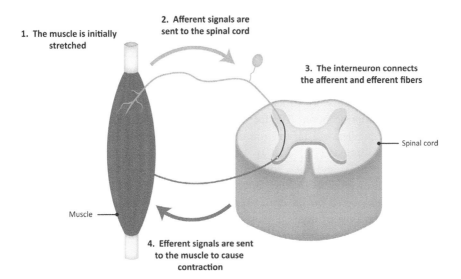

1. The muscle is initially stretched

2. Afferent signals are sent to the spinal cord

3. The interneuron connects the afferent and efferent fibers

Spinal cord

Muscle

4. Efferent signals are sent to the muscle to cause contraction

FIGURE 4.2 Tendon or myotactic reflex with monosynaptic excitation of the agonist muscle and disynaptic reciprocal inhibition of the antagonist muscle (reciprocal inhibition not shown in this figure)

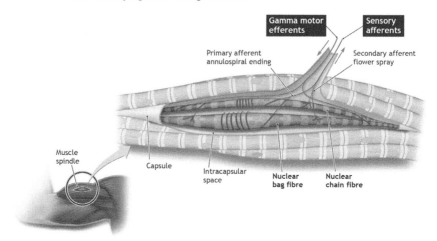

FIGURE 4.3 Nuclear bag and chain fibres located within an intrafusal muscle spindle

to reduce resistance to the walking movement. However, if you are sprinting and the hamstrings get stretched or elongated to a great extent, they also will be subjected to myotactic reflexes to protect them from being extended too far.

Within the muscle spindle, there are nuclear chain fibres that preferentially respond to changes in the amount of stretch or elongation of the muscle, whereas the nuclear bag fibres respond to both the extent and the rate of elongation (Figure 4.3). When activated, nuclear chain and bag fibre impulses are sent to the spinal motoneurons via annulospiral (high conduction velocity) and flower-spray endings (low conduction velocity) through Ia (nuclear bag and chains) and II (nuclear chains) afferents, respectively. As previously mentioned, a monosynaptic myotactic reflex is initiated from the rapid stretch action, resulting in the depolarization/activation (contraction) of the α-motoneuron of the stretched muscle and inhibition (disynaptic) of the antagonist muscle (18).

The spindles also work to inform the system about a body segment's position in space or proprioception. The intensity or discharge rate of the impulses from the muscle spindles will inform the central nervous system about the rate and extent of movement (19). This is why you can close your eyes, abduct and extend your arms, and then still touch your nose. Your muscle spindles are informing the system about how fast and far you have moved in order to reach your nose and, based on previous experience, when to slow down and stop so you do not break your nose.

Another receptor that is activated by tension exerted on the muscle tendon and muscle is the GTO (Figure 4.4) (20,21). The GTO receptors within the tendon are shaped like coiled elastics and, when they are uncoiled due to tension, a piezo-electric effect occurs. Certain biological materials such as crystals (bone), proteins, DNA, and others can discharge an electrical charge in response to mechanical stress (22). Piezo-electricity means electricity resulting from pressure,

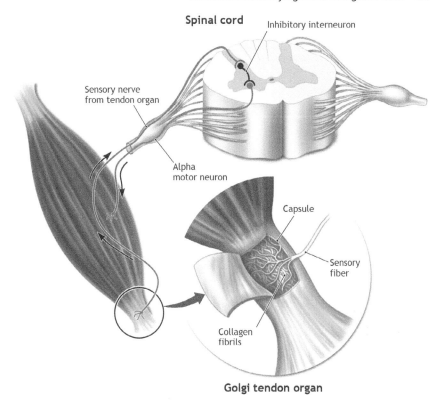

FIGURE 4.4   Golgi tendon organs

derived from the Greek *piezō* or *piezein*, which means to squeeze or press. So, when a contraction occurs or tension is exerted on the musculotendinous unit, the GTO discharges signals to the central nervous system. Although the GTO can reflexively excite the system, under these circumstances it typically results in an inhibitory signal which is labelled as an autogenic inhibition. This reflex is disynaptic in that the GTO synapses with an inhibitory interneuron in the spinal cord, which then inhibits the same muscle group that experienced the tension (23). Although theoretically the GTO should contribute to stretch-induced reflex inhibition, Edin and Vallbo (24) found that, although most spindle afferents respond rapidly to stretch, GTOs were insensitive to the tension produced on the tendon with stretch. If there is a stretch-induced GTO inhibition, it is more likely to occur with large amplitude stretches (7). Furthermore, any possible GTO inhibition subsides almost immediately (60–100 ms post-stretching) after the stretching discontinues (21).

Together with the GTO inhibition to large amplitude stretches, the Renshaw cells can also play a minor role with large amplitude stretches. Renshaw cell inhibition is also known as recurrent inhibition (Figure 4.5). Recurrent or Renshaw cell inhibition can exert stabilizing effects on motoneuron discharge

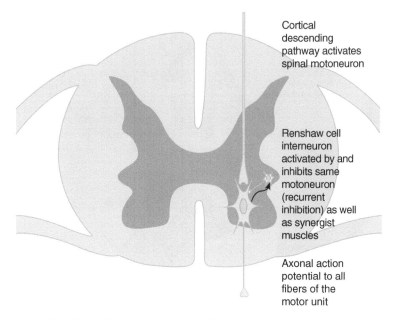

Cortical descending pathway activates spinal motoneuron

Renshaw cell interneuron activated by and inhibits same motoneuron (recurrent inhibition) as well as synergist muscles

Axonal action potential to all fibers of the motor unit

FIGURE 4.5 Renshaw cells and recurrent inhibition

variability and motor unit synchronization during voluntary muscle contractions (25). Recurrent inhibition is more prevalent with weak than with strong contractions, and phasic rather than tonic contractions (26). As the stress or tension on the muscle during a large amplitude stretch is still much less than with a maximal contraction, it should contribute to motoneuron inhibition and muscle relaxation. However, as it is more prevalent with phasic contractions, it may play a more predominant role with full ROM dynamic stretching compared with lesser effects with static stretching.

We have discussed the possible roles of nuclear chain and bag fibres of the muscle spindles, Renshaw cells, and GTOs. Cutaneous nerve fibres can also contribute to the ROM capabilities (Figure 4.6). Cutaneous receptors have polysynaptic innervations to motoneurons and are monitored with the extero-ceptive reflex (E-reflex). Research has demonstrated that small-amplitude passive stretches induce pre-synaptic inhibition (e.g. decreased H-reflex) but no change in the E-reflex (cutaneous) (27) or corticospinal excitability, as measured with motor-evoked potentials (MEPs) induced by transcranial magnetic stimulation (TMS). However, with a greater ROM, both H- and E-reflexes decreased similarly, suggesting that post-synaptic inhibitory mechanisms contribute to the observed changes, but they persist only for a few seconds after completion of the stretching. According to Guissard and Duchateau (7), joint and cutaneous receptors are not significant inhibitors, with small-amplitude stretches, and only a small contribution during large-amplitude stretches.

Cutaneous Receptors

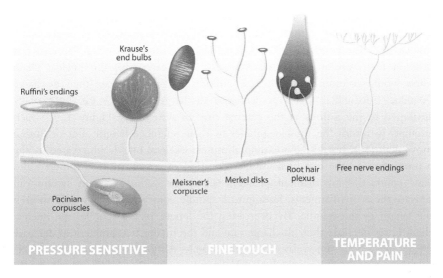

FIGURE 4.6 Cutaneous nerve receptors

With an active static stretch, the individual will use another muscle group – typically, the antagonist muscles to help move the target muscle and joint through an extended ROM. For example, to stretch the hamstrings, you may actively contract quadriceps to flex the hip, which will naturally extend the hamstring muscles that work as hip extensors. Reciprocal inhibition (28,29) may play a role in this situation because quadriceps contraction changes the length of the quadriceps muscle spindles at a particular rate, and can lead to an inhibitory disynaptic reflex synapse with its antagonist, whereas the hamstrings lead to more relaxation.

So, let's go through a static stretching scenario of a person who is lying on their back (supine position); in the first instance, a partner flexes the hip of their extended leg towards their chest to stretch the hamstrings and, in the second, the person contracts their quadriceps and uses their arms to pull their extended leg towards their chest. In the passive static stretching situation of the first scenario, the muscles spindles, specifically the nuclear bag fibres, would detect a slow-to-moderate rate of muscle length change, whereas the nuclear chain fibres would predominately monitor the extent of change in muscle length. Both nuclear bag and chain fibres would discharge at a relatively high frequency with annulospiral and flower-spray ending through the Ia and II afferent nerve trunks, to initiate the myotactic reflexes and cause contractions of the hamstrings, thus resisting stretching of the muscle. In one study, although participants were instructed to relax during a dorsiflexor stretch, electromyographic (EMG) activity reached 5.5% and 8.5% of a maximal voluntary contraction (MVC) in the gastrocnemius and soleus muscles, respectively (30). Therefore, muscle spindle reflexes would have contributed to the "passive" resistance of the musculotendinous unit during the stretch.

Naturally, once the stretch had reached the maximum ROM, there would no longer be any change in the rate of stretch. Within seconds, the nuclear bag fibres would begin to decrease their discharge rate, hence decreasing the intensity of the myotactic reflex contractions (disfacilitation). As the stretch was held in this position for a prolonged period (typically 15–60 seconds), the nuclear chain fibres would accommodate this new position and also decrease their discharge frequency (disfacilitation). This decreased discharge frequency can be partially attributed to the actions of the gamma-efferent system (see Figure 4.3), which attempts to return the muscle spindles to their reference length after or during movement (17). Just like the extrafusal muscle (skeletal muscle innervated by the α-motoneuron), the intrafusal muscles (location of sensory muscle spindles) also have contractile myofilament proteins. Thus, the gamma-efferent system can activate these myofilaments, leading to a spindle contraction that would shorten the length of the spindle. By decreasing the length of the spindle, the nuclear chain fibres decrease their discharge rate and the myotactic contractions decrease further, leading to more relaxation of the muscle. Although elongating the muscle to the end of ROM would have placed tension on the GTOs which should activate greater type Ib afferent inhibitory stimulation, there is little evidence that it contributes to substantial muscle relaxation (perhaps a small contribution with an extensive ROM to maximal point of discomfort). Try this yourself. Stretch any muscle passively and hold it for 30 seconds or more. Then see if you can stretch the muscle or increase the ROM further. It is guaranteed that you will have a greater ROM. If you used an active static stretch then the contraction of quadriceps may have also contributed to further relaxation with the reciprocal inhibition effect.

So, which process is more predominant with static stretching – inhibition or disfacilitation? In one study H- and T-reflexes were compared in soleus with increases in ankle ROM (31). The H-reflex amplitude decreased more than the T-reflex one (31% vs 8% of control). When the stretching was completed, the H-reflex returned immediately to its control value, whereas the T-reflex remained depressed. Therefore, the T-reflex reduction was more probably derived from either a decrease in muscle spindle sensitivity (disfacilitation) or increased musculotendinous unit compliance (mechanical change). According to this study, during the stretch there could be pre-synaptic inhibition and muscle spindle-induced disfacilitation of the motoneuron, whereas the persistent increases in ROM would be attributed more to spindle disfacilitation and perhaps muscu-lotendinous compliance. In fact, we can go even deeper than that. Are there differences in how the muscle reflexes are inhibited if you have a small- versus a large-amplitude stretch? It has been shown that passive small-amplitude stretches decrease the H-reflex through pre-synaptic inhibition. The pre-synaptic Ia inhibition pathway originates from the intrafusal muscle spindle fibres and projects pre-synaptically (before the junction of the dendrite and the motoneuron) by interneurons on to the Ia terminals (32). Thus, there is no intrinsic change in motoneuron excitability. With larger-amplitude passive stretches, there may be suppression of the cortical neurons and α-motoneuron excitability (32). In this case with large-amplitude stretches, GTO's inhibitory afferents could contribute to decreased motoneuron excitability from Ib fibres (32). GTOs respond primarily to muscle contraction forces, but are not very sensitive to the degree of force or stress associated with smaller-amplitude passive stretching (32). Remember, however, that GTO effects would continue only during the period of stretch and tend to diminish rapidly thereafter (21). There is also the possibility of post-synaptic inhibition with large-amplitude stretches from the inhibitory effect of the Renshaw cell recurrent inhibition loop (33).

It is, in fact, possible that stretch-induced reflex interneuron inhibition might affect not only the muscles being stretched but also distant or non-local muscles. There are a few studies that have demonstrated that stretching the hamstrings unilaterally (only one side of the body) will improve ROM of the contralateral (opposite side) hamstrings (34). Our lab has also shown that static or dynamic stretching of the shoulders will increase ROM of the hamstrings, whereas stretching the hip adductor (groin) muscles increased the flexibility of the shoulders (35). This research could be crucial evidence for the pervasive effects of stretch-induced neural inhibition that acts globally on the body.

Neural mechanisms of acute PNF stretching

Traditionally, PNF was considered more effective than static stretching for increasing ROM due to the variety of reflex inhibition techniques that were proposed to be involved. For example, with the CRAC (contract–relax agonist–contract) method, the muscle to be stretched (e.g. hamstrings) would be actively placed in an elongated position by contracting the antagonist muscle (e.g. hip flexion by quadriceps), which would activate reciprocal inhibition. Reciprocal inhibition is a reflex branch of the myotactic reflex. As a reminder, the myotactic reflex is a monosynaptic reflex initiated from the stretching of the muscle spindles, resulting in an excitation of the stretched muscle. This muscle spindle-induced excitation also has an afferent nerve branch that excites an inhibitory interneuron which suppresses the activity of an antagonist motoneuron (disynaptic). In this example, contracting quadriceps to lengthen the hamstrings would change the length of many quadriceps muscle spindles (especially in the distal regions), causing further excitation of quadriceps with inhibition of the hamstrings, permitting greater muscle excursion (elongation). The next step with CRAC PNF stretching would be to contract the stretched muscle (e.g. hamstrings) against a partner's resistance or it can also be against an immovable object such as a wall. This contraction, which does not need to be a maximal contraction, because Roger Enoka (a very prominent and internationally renowned neuromuscular scientist) and colleagues (12) found that, whether the contraction was performed at 50 or 100% of the participants' maximal voluntary force, there was a similar reduction in the H-reflex amplitude (afferent excitability of the α-motoneuron). Furthermore, this contraction of an elongated muscle would place stress on the GTO, possibly leading to its activation inducing autogenic inhibition (36). Autogenic inhibition from GTO activation increases Ib muscle afferent activity (21), which hyperpolarizes the dendrites synapsing with spinal α-motoneurons of the stretched muscle, decreasing or blocking the Ia afferent reflex activity and enabling further increases in ROM (20). However, there is no direct evidence for a positive relationship between the aforementioned reflex activity and PNF ROM (20). One might expect this reciprocal and autogenic reflex inhibition to decrease muscle activity, as evidenced by attenuated EMG activity, but a number of studies have illustrated increased resting EMG activity immediately after the contraction phase of a PNF stretch (37,38). As GTO effects persist briefly after tension to the receptors has been removed (39), the autogenic inhibition effects should not persist and their contribution to PNF flexibility is highly debatable (36,40). Although depression of the spinal reflex excitability after the isometric contraction is brief (<5 s), it could still persist long enough to provide an advantage for the subsequent stretch. Thus, similar to static stretching, there could be some reflex inhibition during the stretching procedure. An increased stretch tolerance (41), decreased viscoelasticity, and a degree of reduced musculotendinous stiffness (37,42) could all contribute to the sustained increase in elastic ROM.

Neural mechanisms of acute dynamic stretching

Whereas static and PNF stretching should reduce muscle activation through some degree of reflexive disfacilitation with reduced muscle spindle receptor activity of the nuclear bag and nuclear chain (Ia afferents) and further possible inhibition from autogenic (Ib afferents) and reciprocal inhibition (Ia afferents), dynamic stretching should excite or increase activation of the system. The previously discussed myotactic reflex activity would be increased by dynamic stretching due to nuclear bag and chain excitation as a result of the higher rate and extent of muscle elongation. As dynamic muscle stretching is usually performed as a relaxed action with submaximal muscle contractions, the activation of GTOs initiating autogenic inhibition would not be expected to play a major role in increasing acute ROM. Reciprocal inhibition would be activated by the sequential movement of the limbs, similar to the well-documented reciprocal inhibition sequences found with locomotor activities such as walking and running (43,44). This reciprocal inhibition could contribute to greater dynamic movement excursions during the stretching activity, but would not persist after the activity. Hence, for the augmentation of ROM to persist after the dynamic stretching, the reciprocal inhibition would need to contribute to viscous and morphological changes, which would continue for a prolonged period after the stretching. Typically, dynamic stretching is not as uncomfortable or painful as static or PNF stretching, hence the role of stretch tolerance may not be as predominant.

Stretch tolerance sensory theory

Increases in ROM could also be attributed to a psycho-physiological effect (sensory theory). Magnusson and colleagues suggest that increased flexibility can be largely attributed to an increased stretch tolerance (45,46). They showed that, after 3 weeks of stretch training, the increased ROM was not attributed to differences in muscle stiffness or reflex EMG activity (45). Increased stretch tolerance could be related to changes in the sensitivity of nociceptive (pain) nerve endings (47), which allow the individual to accommodate greater discomfort or pain and thus push themselves through a greater ROM. Passive stretching can produce acute ischaemic compression, which has been shown to result in reduced perceived pain in the neck and shoulder muscles (48). Freitas et al. (49), in a meta-analysis, examined 26 stretch-training studies that ranged from 3 weeks to 8 weeks in duration, with a weekly stretching duration of 1165 seconds per week (about 20 minutes). Stretching for 3–8 weeks did not, on average, alter muscle and tendon properties, and thus the increased extensibility must have been related to a greater tolerance to tension. However, if stretch tolerance was the only mechanism at play with no substantial reflex inhibition occurring, then the commonly found static stretch-induced performance impairments would not be expected from non-stretched muscles.

However, we not only found that stretching one muscle can increase the ROM of another muscle but also reported that unilateral static stretching of the plantar flexors (calf muscles) led to impairments of jump height in the contralateral lower limb (50), and stretching the shoulders also impaired lower limb jump performance (51). Static stretching of the pectoralis major muscle decreased activation of triceps brachii during a bench-press action (52). There are not many questions in the world that are simply black and white. So, although an increased stretch tolerance (totally psychological or psycho-physiological influenced by type III and IV nociceptor afferents) can certainly help explain ROM improvements, it seems likely that some degree of afferent stretch-induced reflex inhibition is also acting on the muscle under stretch, as well as other non-affected muscles. Although this reflex inhibition would be most predominant during the holding of the stretch, the reported subsequent impairments in non-local jump performance and muscle activation suggest that it can persist for a few minutes after stretching. However, even if neural reflex inhibition works primarily during the actual stretching exercise, permitting a greater elongation of the muscle, it might impact morphological structures such as muscles, tendons, and in some cases ligaments.

Acute morphological static stretching mechanisms

Greater stretch tolerance or neural inhibition should allow the muscle to be elongated to a greater degree. Maintaining this greater elongation over an extended period (i.e. 20–60 seconds) might be expected to affect the properties of the musculotendinous tissues. What musculoskeletal components restrict our ROM? ROM is affected by skeletal structures, joint capsules, ligaments, muscles, tendons, aponeuroses, and fat. What factors can we modify with stretching? If we stretch until a bone is fractured, we can get an acute increase in ROM but at the cost of excessive pain, inflammation, and loss of function. Within moments, the pain and inflammation will then decrease the ROM! The glenoid fossa or cavity of the shoulder (glenohumeral) joint is a relatively flat surface, allowing the shoulder a great deal of unrestricted movement for flexion/extension, abduction/adduction, horizontal abduction/adduction, medial and lateral rotation, and circumduction (Figure 4.7a). In contrast, the acetabulum of the hip joint is deeper and more cup-like, restricting ROM compared with the glenoid fossa (Figure 4.7b). It can also perform flexion/extension, abduction/adduction, medial and lateral rotation and circumduction. Whereas shoulder motion is expansive, hip ROM is quite limited compared with the shoulder.

Shoulder Anatomy

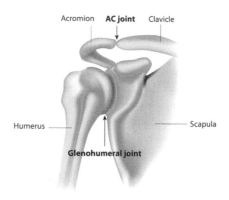

The Hip Joint

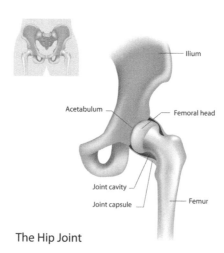

FIGURE 4.7   Skeletal restrictions on ROM

Normal ROM	Hip (°)	Shoulder (°)
Flexion	110–120	180
Extension	10–15	45–60
Abduction	30–50	150
External rotation (lateral)	40–60	90
Internal rotation (medial)	30–40	70–90

Thus, skeletal structures are typically not modifiable with any amount or type of warm-up and stretching will typically not affect the skeletal structures.

Ligaments are tough fibrous tissue which connects one bone to another bone, providing joint stability. An important function is to prevent movement that might damage a joint. In most circumstances, the objective of stretching is NOT to elongate the ligaments. Lengthening ligaments would decrease joint stability and often lead to injury. There are some cases, however, when the goal of stretching would be to elongate ligaments. Athletes who need to attain extreme levels of flexibility such as gymnasts, figure skaters, dancers, certain circus performers, and others may target their ligaments.

Some individuals have a predisposition to hyperlaxity of their connective tissue or hypermobility of their joints. Women tend to have greater joint laxity or hypermobility compared with men (53–57). Harry Houdini (1874–1926) was famous for his escape abilities (Figure 4.8). He could be tied up in ropes or chains and submerged in water or other hazards (i.e. suspended from buildings) and would make miraculous escapes. Houdini had lax ligaments and could subluxate (partially dislocate) or dislocate many of his joints. Hence, movements that were impossible for the average individual were possible for Houdini by voluntarily subluxating a joint, sliding or moving out of a chain or rope, and then popping the joint back into place before reappearing before the audience. Naturally, you should not need to be warned that you should not try this at home. Average individuals who experience an injury with a joint dislocation or subluxation often have difficulties throughout their life with subsequent dislocations. People with hypermobile joints (Figure 4.9) can experience increased chances for nerve compression disorders (58), impaired proprioception (59,60), and increased risk of joint trauma and osteoarthritis (61–63). Ligaments lack the extensive vascularity of muscles and tendons and tend not to heal or recover completely back to their original length and tension. So, unless there is a need for extreme ROM capabilities by an athlete, stretching for health and normal function should not be so severe as to lengthen the ligaments (includes joint capsule). However, placing mechanical stress on ligaments, as with stretching, can play an important role in the processes of cellular differentiation up-regulating (increasing the activity of) ligament fibroblast markers such as collagen types I and III and tenascin-C (64). Thus stretch-induced mechanical stress would help build the ligament matrix, making it stronger and more resistant to damage or injury.

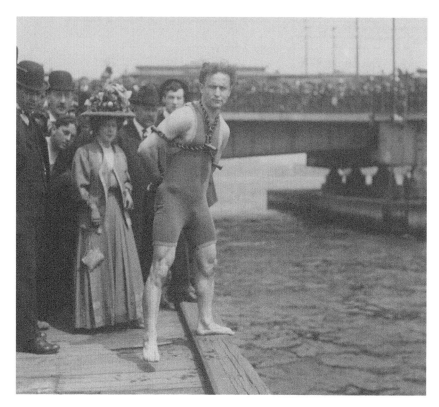

FIGURE 4.8 Harry Houdini

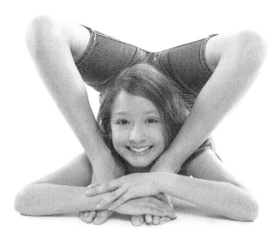

FIGURE 4.9 Contortionist with hypermobile joints

Similar effects are seen with tendon tissue, where a lack of mechanical stress can cause a progressive loss of cell matrix, and a prolonged period of stress deprivation results in the even higher mechanical stresses needed to promote tendon tissue growth than before the removal of stress strain (65).

Excessive fat can affect flexibility tests. An abundance of adiposity around the waist and trunk will impede hip flexion, for example, although there is no concrete evidence that fat will impede the extensibility of tissues. An early study by Tyrance (66), did not find any significant correlation between low-fat, high-fat and muscular individuals, and their flexibility. Alter (15) points out that very large sumo wrestlers with an overabundance of fat can still exhibit extraordinary levels of flexibility. Of course, fat is not a tissue targeted during the stretching of a warm-up. Proper diet and exercise are the key to improving fat-induced restrictions on some ROM tests (i.e. sit and reach or toe touch).

When stretching, can we elongate the nerves? Nerves do have the capacity to elongate to a certain point. The extensibility of the nerve resides mostly with the perineurium (connective tissue sheath surrounding a bundle [fascicle] of nerve fibres within a nerve), with an elongation range between 6% and 20% of its resting length (15,67,68). Once the maximum length has been reached, the nerve is susceptible to tearing or injury. If the perineurium or nerve is ruptured, there can be leakage of proteins into the fascicles, and oedema and reduced possibility for regeneration (69). Furthermore, stretching the nerve as much as 8% can reduce blood flow with complete occlusion at 15% elongation (70–72). Nerve conduction can also be inhibited with only 6% elongation (69,73). As long as the maximum elongation limit is not exceeded, then the nerve should be able to return to its original length (74). With muscle fascicles able to elongate approximately 50%, how is it possible that we can stretch without always damaging our nerves? Although the nerve itself can only elongate 6–20%, the nerves are not typically situated in a straight line but are rather in a slacker position due to an undulating path through the tissues (fasciculi) (75). So, when stretching, the nerve does not initially elongate, but it actually straightens out until there is no longer an undulating course. Thus, we can stretch far greater lengths than 20% of the resting length of the musculotendinous tissues without damaging the nerves. Another evolutionary safety aspect is that most nerves traverse the flexor side of the joint. When a joint is flexed, the nerves would actually be placed in a more relaxed position rather than under the stress of an elongated position. Exceptions to this general rule are the ulnar nerve which traverses the extensor aspect of the elbow. You will experience the anatomical position of your ulnar nerve when you hit your "funny bone" and feel the "humour" of the pain running up your arm because you hit the ulnar nerve near the humerus. The sciatic nerve is another exception to the flexor positioning of nerves because it runs across the extensor aspect of the hip. The sciatic nerve is protected by an especially thick epineurium, which constitutes about 88% of its cross-sectional area (68), because we spend an inordinate amount of time squatting (elongating the nerve tract) and sitting on the sciatic nerve (15). Therefore, elongation of our nerves is not a primary aim of stretching. The primary tissues targeted by stretching are the muscles and tendons.

In the past, strength training resulting in muscle hypertrophy was feared to result in "muscle boundness". Being "muscle bound" inferred having large muscles that would inhibit flexibility. Contrary to this myth, there are examples of hypertrophied bodybuilders such as "Flex Wheeler" who could perform the Russian splits (legs spread laterally or fully abducted) during competitions. There are many other hypertrophied athletes such as American football players, rugby, ice hockey players, sumo wrestlers, and others who exhibit superb levels of flexibility. Although performing partial ROM (also known as cheat "reps"), resistance training can shorten a muscle inhibiting ROM; there are a number of studies demonstrating increased ROM when performing full ROM resistance training (76–80). These resistance training ROM improvements are also seen with senior adults (81,82). Although not every study finds an increase in flexibility with resistance training, there is typically no loss of ROM (83). Thus, large muscles have a great propensity for extensibility.

Muscles have both intracellular and extracellular components. When stretching a muscle, what parts are actually being stretched? Myofibrils can be stretched to twice their resting length without damage (84). The elasticity of the myofibrils is largely due to an intracellular protein called titin, with a length of approximately half the sarcomere being anchored at the Z-disc (through a telethonin protein) and the M-line (Figure 4.10) (84). Titin can act as a spring that unfolds in response to high tension or stress. Myofibrils are connected together by the extracellular matrix. An essential protein in the extracellular matrix is fibronectin, which has elastic properties. Fibronectin can stretch up to four times its resting relaxed length. It is composed of three subunits (FN-I, FN-II, and FM-III), with FN-III as the subunit that unfolds to contribute to the elasticity (Figure 4.11). Stressing these units mechanically, thermally, or chemically leads to further binding with other fragments (e.g. anastellin) to form superfibronectins with increased adhesion capabilities. Fibronectins are also in contact with integrin molecules on the muscle membrane (84), which also sense membrane tension and transfer this infor-mation to the Raptor–mTOR (mammalian target of rapamycin) complex in the nucleus, helping to promote greater protein synthesis (85,86). Specifically, integrin links laminin in the extracellular matrix with the cell cytoskeleton and translates mechanical forces into chemical signals. Stretching and muscle contractions activate intracellular signalling molecules that respond to injury-induced damage. Integrin stabilizes the muscle and provides communication between the matrix and cytoskeleton. Thus, elevated tension from stretching detected by the integrin molecule transduced to the nucleus leads to increased protein synthesis and helps with injury protection and prevention (87).

This enhanced muscle protein synthesis would increase muscle volume and strength, protecting it from other similar force stressors. An animal experiment had

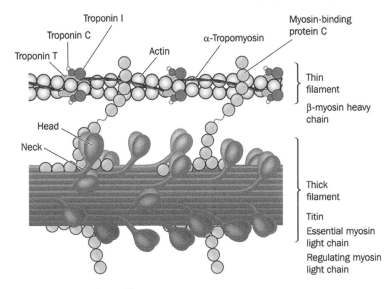

Troponin I

Troponin C

Troponin T

Actin

α-Tropomyosin

Myosin-binding
protein C

Head

Neck

Thin
filament

β-myosin heavy
chain

Thick
filament

Titin

Essential myosin
light chain

Regulating myosin
light chain

FIGURE 4.10 Titin and myofilament structure

chicken latissimus dorsi (lats) muscles passively stretched over an extended duration (days). Fortunately, or unfortunately for the chickens, they were sacrificed and the muscles were used in isolation in a physiological saline bath solution. Researchers found an increase in muscle protein synthesis activity just by passively stretching the isolated muscle (88). Not all animal model experiments transfer easily to humans, and I would not suggest hanging from a bar or being placed on a rack for days or weeks to increase the hypertrophy of your "lats". However, it does demonstrate how the tension from a passive stretch is transduced (signal is sent) by the membrane integrin molecule to the Raptor–mTOR complex in the nucleus, to activate the transcription and translation activities of the DNA to promote muscle growth (increased protein synthesis). This stretch-induced adaptation may contribute to the increased tolerance of the muscle matrix to external forces and torques, decreasing injury incidence.

Static stretching has often been prescribed as part of a warm-up or a training routine because it is purported to decrease the incidence of musculotendinous injuries (9,89). The rationale for decreased musculotendinous injuries would be that the muscles and tendons would be better able to withstand or absorb the forces placed on the tissues and not tear (muscle strain or tendon sprain). Logically, then, increased ROM should be ascribed to not only decreased viscosity, neural inhibition, and stretch tolerance but also decreased stiffness or increased compliance of the muscles and tendons. There is much conflict in the literature as to the extent of tissue compliance/stiffness changes. Some researchers claim an association between reductions in myotendinous stiffness and ROM after an acute bout of static stretching (90), suggesting that altered muscle mechanical properties are important

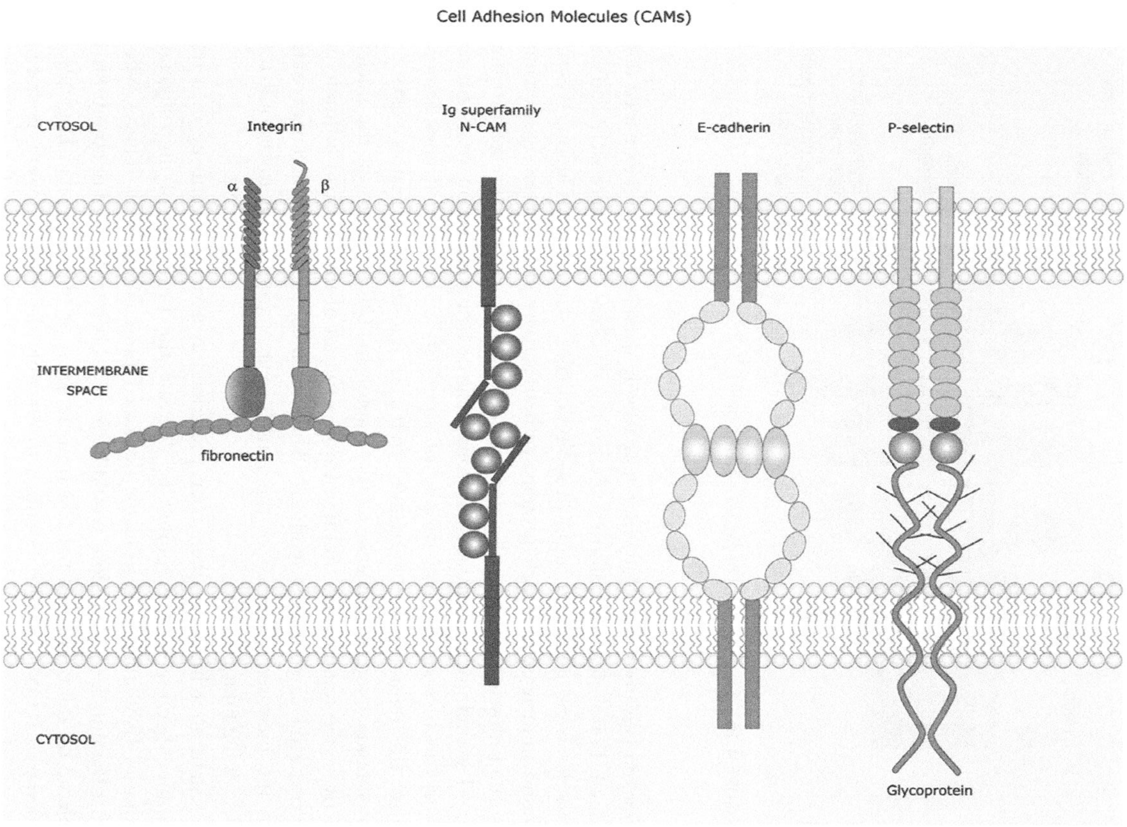

FIGURE 4.11 Fibronectin and integrin

contributors (90). Two very important stretch researchers, Anthony Blazevich (Australia) and Anthony Kay (UK), investigated the contribution of muscle and tendon elongation to the maximum dorsiflexor ROM. They found that muscular tissue is more compliant than the tendon during passive stretch. In their study, muscle lengthened 14.9% compared with 8.4% lengthening of the tendon under maximal stretch conditions (30). Thus, the maximum dorsiflexion ankle ROM was not constrained by tendon elongation because further tendon strain should have been possible. Similarly, Abellaneda (91), from the Guissard and Duchateau lab, indicated that the relative contribution of muscle fascicles to musculotendinous unit elongation was 71.8% whereas the tendon contributed 28.2%. Tendons are composed of 60–85% collagen protein (4), whereas connective tissue in muscle constitutes between 1% and 10%. Collagen is a very strong fibrous tissue, explaining the decreased tendon compliance. It is important to note that these studies show the response of muscle and tendon to stretching. However, before stretching, the resting length of the tendon far exceeds the muscle fascicles and thus the tendon can account for about half of the change in musculotendinous unit length. As tendon elongation exceeds muscle elongation, stress-induced muscle strain surpasses tendon strain by about fourfold (92). Freitas et al. (49), in their meta-analysis of 26 stretch-training studies, found there were trivial effects of stretch training on tendon stiffness, whereas one study actually demonstrated lower tendon extensibility after 3 weeks of stretch training (93). Hence, although tendons contribute greatly to ROM, the lesser elongation of the muscle fascicles causes them to receive more of the strain caused by stretching, thus leading to a greater chance for muscle strains versus tendon sprains.

Another means of increasing muscle length might be to change both the length and the angle of the muscle fascicles (fibres). In the same study by Blazevich et al. (30), they reported that the contribution of changes in fascicle angle to the maximum stretch capabilities was negligible compared with the contributions of fascicle elongation. There is also a minor contribution to increased muscle elongation from fascicle rotation. A significant difference between flexible and inflexible individuals is that fascicle rotation during stretch was greater in flexible (~40% at 30° dorsiflexion) than inflexible individuals (~25%) (30). Thus, rotation permits interfascicle (and interfibre) translation. As little difference has been reported between flexible and inflexible individuals in muscle lengthening and changes in fascicle length (series elastic component), the significant differences in fascicle rotation suggest a substantial difference in the parallel elastic component as well as the previously reported greater stretch tolerances of flexible individuals.

Acute morphological PNF stretching mechanisms

Similar morphological mechanisms might be expected with PNF stretching. Static stretching is reported to be more effective in decreasing muscle stiffness (94), whereas PNF is more efficient in reducing both muscle and tendon stiffness (42). Perhaps, as PNF is reported to increase stretch tolerance more than static stretching (94), the higher stretch tolerance may provide greater stress on both the muscle and the tendon. It might be rationalized that the contractions employed with contract–relax (CR) and CRAC PNF stretching provides a mental distraction (95), permitting a greater pain or stretch tolerance. As mentioned previously, the literature is conflicted as to whether PNF actually provides greater (96–99), similar (100,101), or trivial (102) increases in ROM compared with static stretching, or even less flexibility than static stretching (103).

Acute morphological dynamic stretching mechanisms

As dynamic stretching uses repeated cyclical loading and unloading of the involved muscles, usually for a few minutes (104), these muscular contractions should induce shear stresses between muscle fibres and increase muscle temperature, decreasing viscosity (thixotropy). In animal models, repeated lengthening and shortening of a muscle has increased muscle extensibility (105). One human dynamic stretching study indicates passive muscle stiffness reductions with increased ROM (106).

Dynamic ballistic stretching has often not been advocated for efficiently improving ROM. Higher-velocity dynamic stretching (ballistic) can weaken tissue (107,108) by producing greater tensile forces over a brief duration (109). These high forces within a short time period do not allow for stress relaxation or creep to occur. Stress relaxation and creep refer to the reduction in tension and tissue-lengthening, respectively, that occur when a tissue is held in a lengthened position for an extended period of time (15). Hence, these mechanisms may explain why ballistic stretching is often found not to provide substantial increases in ROM, and the fear that ballistic stretching is more likely to lead to injuries especially with muscle that is not warmed up. Unfortunately, there is limited literature rationalizing the ROM morphological mechanisms for dynamic stretching.

Summary

Increased flexibility can be achieved even without stretching. Increasing tissue (muscles and tendons) temperatures elicit thixotropic effects, which decrease tissue viscoelasticity. Static and PNF stretching can activate a number of inhibitory reflexes. Prolonged static modes of stretching can disfacilitate spindle reflexes as well as inducing pre- and post-synaptic inhibition of the afferents. Specifically, the activity (discharge frequency) of intrafusal, muscle spindle, nuclear chain (detects extent of stretch), and nuclear bag (detects the extent and rate of stretch) fibres diminishes with the static modes of stretching. Although GTOs are predominately inhibitory, they do not respond strongly to stretch and any extent of inhibition from GTOs subside almost immediately after the stretch. Furthermore, Renshaw cells also do not play a substantial inhibitory role with static stretching. However, extensive static stretching can activate cutaneous afferent inhibition. Active static and PNF stretching, which involve the contraction of the antagonist muscle, could initiate the contribution of reciprocal inhibition. PNF stretching also uses many of these inhibitory mechanisms, whereas dynamic stretching tends to excite rather than inhibit these reflexes. Hence, the stretch tolerance theory can also help explain increased ROM as the individual accommodates the discomfort or pain associated with stretching and can push themselves past their previous ROM.

Morphological considerations include the skeletal configuration and alignment that cannot be modified with stretching. Ligaments that help secure bone to bone (joint stability) are primarily inelastic and avascular, and thus are also resistant to elastic or plastic elongation by stretching, except with the intense flexibility training routines of extreme athletes such as gymnasts, dancers, figure skaters, and others. Excessive fat can impede joint ROM. Nerves can acutely elongate approximately 6–20% of their resting length but thereafter they are susceptible to injury. Highly hypertrophied muscle can also provide some ROM restrictions; however, the great extensibility of muscle puts into dispute the old theory of muscle boundness. Myofibrils can elongate to double their resting length mainly due to the protein titin. Muscle is more compliant than tendons, with tendons accounting for less than half of the musculotendinous unit change. Muscle extensibility can also be altered by changes in fascicle angle (trivial), fascicle rotation (minor), and fascicle elongation (substantial). However, stretch tolerance may provide a greater impetus to enhanced ROM than decreased musculotendinous stiffness.

References

1. Young WB. The use of static stretching in warm-up for training and competition. *Int J Sports Physiol Perform* 2: 212–216, 2007.
2. Young WB and Behm DG. Effects of running, static stretching and practice jumps on explosive force production and jumping performance. *J Sports Med Phys Fitness* 43: 21–27, 2003.
3. Smith NP, Barclay CJ, and Loiselle DS. The efficiency of muscle contraction. *Prog Biophys Mol Biol* 88: 1–58, 2005.
4. Kjaer M. Role of extracellular matrix in adaptation of tendon and skeletal muscle to mechanical loading. *Physiol Rev* 84: 649–698, 2004.
5. Drinkwater EJ and Behm DG. Effects of 22 degrees C muscle temperature on voluntary and evoked muscle properties during and after high-intensity exercise. *Appl Physiol Nutr Metab* 32: 1043–1051, 2007.
6. Faulkner JA, Zerba E, and Brooks SV. Muscle temperature of mammals: Cooling impairs most functional properties. *Am J Physiol* 259: R259–R265, 1990.
7. Guissard N and Duchateau J. Neural aspects of muscle stretching. *Exerc Sport Sci Rev* 34: 154–158, 2006.
8. Behm DG, Bambury A, Cahill F, and Power K. Effect of acute static stretching on force, balance, reaction time, and movement time. *Med Sci Sports Exerc* 36: 1397–1402, 2004.

9. Behm DG, Blazevich AJ, Kay AD, and McHugh M. Acute effects of muscle stretching on physical performance, range of motion, and injury incidence in healthy active individuals: A systematic review. *Appl Physiol Nutr Metab* 41: 1–11, 2016.

10. Behm DG, Button DC, and Butt JC. Factors affecting force loss with prolonged stretching. *Can J Appl Physiol* 26: 261–272, 2001.

11. Behm DG and Chaouachi A. A review of the acute effects of static and dynamic stretching on performance. *Eur J Appl Physiol* 111: 2633–2651, 2011.

12. Enoka RM, Hutton RS, and Eldred E. Changes in excitability of tendon tap and Hoffmann reflexes following voluntary contractions. *Electroencephalogr Clin Neurophysiol* 48: 664–672, 1980.

13. Timofeev I, Grenier F, and Steriade M. Disfacilitation and active inhibition in the neocortex during the natural sleep-wake cycle: An intracellular study. *Proc Natl Acad Sci USA* 98: 1924–1929, 2001.

14. Avela J, Kyrïlñinen H, and Komi PV. Altered reflex sensitivity after repeated and prolonged passive muscle stretching. *J Appl Physiol* 86: 1283–1291, 1999.

15. Alter MJ. *Science of Flexibility*. Champaign, IL: Human Kinetics, 1996.

16. Matthews PBC. Developing views on the muscle spindle. In: *Spinal and Supraspinal Mechanisms of Voluntary Motor Control and Locomotion*. JE Desmedt, ed. Basel: Karger, 1980, pp 12–27.

17. Matthews PBC. Muscle spindles: their messages and their fusimotor supply. In: *The Nervous System: Handbook of Physiology*. VB Brooks, ed. Rockville, MA: American Physiological Society, 1981, pp 189–288.

18. McArdle WD, Katch FI, and Katch VL. *Exercise Physiology: Energy, Nutrition, and Human Performance*. Malvern, PA: Lea & Febiger, 1991.

19. Proske U. What is the role of muscle receptors in proprioception? *Muscle & Nerve* 31: 780–787, 2005.

20. Chalmers G. Re-examination of the possible role of Golgi tendon organ and muscle spindle reflexes in proprioceptive neuromuscular facilitation muscle stretching. *Sports Biomech* 3: 159–183, 2004.

21. Houk JC, Crago PE, and Rymer WZ. Functional properties of the Golgi tendon organs. In: *Spinal and Supraspinal Mechanisms of Voluntary Motor Control and Locomotion*. JE Desmedt, ed. Basel: Karger, 1980, pp 33–43.

22. Shamos MH and Lavine LS. Piezoelectricity as a fundamental property of biological tissues. *Nature* 213: 267–269, 1967.

23. Khan SI and Burne JA. Afferents contributing to autogenic inhibition of gastrocnemius following electrical stimulation of its tendon. *Brain Res* 1282: 28–37, 2009.

24. Edin BB and Vallbo AB. Classification of human muscle stretch receptor afferents: A Bayesian approach. *J Neurophysiol* 63: 1314–1322, 1990.

25. Mattei B, Schmied A, Mazzocchio R, Decchi B, Rossi A, and Vedel JP. Pharmacologically induced enhancement of recurrent inhibition in humans: Effects on motoneurone discharge patterns. *J Physiol* 548: 615–629, 2003.

26. Katz R and Pierrot-Deseilligny E. Recurrent inhibition in humans. *Prog Neurobiol* 57: 325–355, 1999.

27. Delwaide PJ, Toulouse P, and Crenna P. Hypothetical role of long-loop reflex pathways. *Appl Neurophysiol* 44: 171–176, 1981.

28. Crone C and Nielson J. Spinal mechanisms in man contributing to reciprocal inhibition during voluntary dorsiflexion of the foot. *J Physiol (Lond)* 116: 255–272, 1989.

29. Petersen N, Morita H, and Nielsen J. Evaluation of reciprocal inhibition of the soleus H-reflex during tonic plantar flexion in man. *J Neurosci Methods* 84: 1–8, 1998.

30. Blazevich AJ, Cannavan D, Waugh CM, Fath F, Miller SC, and Kay AD. Neuromuscular factors influencing the maximum stretch limit of the human plantar flexors. *J Appl Physiol* 113: 1446–1455, 2012.

31. Guissard N, Duchateau J, and Hainaut K. Muscle stretching and motoneuron excitability. *Eur J Appl Physiol* 58: 47–52, 1988.

32. Guissard N, Duchateau J, and Hainaut K. Mechanisms of decreased motoneurone excitation during passive muscle stretching. *Exp Brain Res* 137: 163–169, 2001.

33. Bussel B and Pierrot-Deseilligny E. Inhibition of human motoneurons, probably of Renshaw origin, elicited by an orthodromic motor discharge. *J Physiol* 269: 319–339, 1977.

34. Chaouachi A, Padulo J, Kasmi S, Othmen AB, Chatra M, and Behm DG. Unilateral static and dynamic hamstrings stretching increases contralateral hip flexion range of motion. *Clin Physiol Funct I* 37 (1): 23–29, 2015.

35. Behm DG, Cavanaugh T, Quigley P, Reid JC, Nardi PS, and Marchetti PH. Acute bouts of upper and lower body static and dynamic stretching increase non-local joint range of motion. *Eur J Appl Physiol* 116: 241–249, 2016.

36. Hindle KBW, Whitcomb TJ, Briggs, WO, and Hong, J. Proprioceptive neuromuscular facilitation (PNF): Its mechanisms and effects on range of motion and muscular function. *J Hum Kinet* 31: 105–113, 2012.

37. Magnusson SP, Simonsen EB, Aagaard P, Dyhre-Poulsen P, McHugh MP, and Kjaer M. Mechanical and physical responses to stretching with and without preisometric contraction in human skeletal muscle. *Arch Phys Med Rehabil* 77: 373–378, 1996.

38. Mitchell UH, Myrer JW, Hopkins JT, Hunter I, Feland JB, and Hilton SC. Neurophysiological reflex mechanisms' lack of contribution to the success of PNF stretches. *J Sport Rehabil* 18: 343–357, 2009.

39. Trajano GS, Nosaka K, and Blazevich AJ. Neurophysiological mechanisms underpinning stretch-induced force loss. *Sports Med* 47 (8): 1531–1541, 2017.

40. Sharman MJ, Cresswell AG, and Riek S. Proprioceptive neuromuscular facilitation stretching: Mechanisms and clinical implications. *Sports Med* 36: 929–939, 2006.

41. Mitchell UH, Myrer JW, Hopkins JT, Hunter I, Feland JB, and Hilton SC. Acute stretch perception alteration contributes to the success of the PNF "contract-relax" stretch. *J Sport Rehabil* 16: 85–92, 2007.

42. Kay AD, Husbands-Beasley J, and Blazevich AJ. Effects of contract-relax, static stretching, and isometric contractions on muscle-tendon mechanics. *Med Sci Sports Exerc* 47: 2181–2190, 2015.

43. Petersen N, Morita H, and Nielsen J. Modulation of reciprocal inhibition between ankle extensors and flexors during walking in man. *J Physiol* 520: 605–619, 1999.

44. Pyndt H, Laursen M, and Nielsen J. Changes in reciprocal inhibition across the ankle joint with changes in external load and pedaling rate during bicycling. *J Neurophysiol* 90: 3168–3177, 2003.

45. Magnusson SP, Simonsen EB, Aagaard P, Sorensen H, and Kjaer M. A mechanism for altered flexibility in human skeletal muscle. *J Physiol* 497 (Pt 1): 291–298, 1996.

46. Magnusson SP, Simonsen EB, Dyhre-Poulsen P, Aagaard P, Mohr T, and Kjaer M. Viscoelastic stress relaxation during static stretch in human skeletal muscle in the absence of EMG activity. *Scand J Med Sci Sports* 6: 323–328, 1996.

47. Marchettini P. Muscle pain: animal and human experimental and clinical studies. *Muscle Nerve* 16: 1033–1039, 1993.

48. Hanten WP, Olson SL, Butts NL, and Nowicki AL. Effectiveness of a home program of ischemic pressure followed by sustained stretch for treatment of myofascial trigger points. *Phys Ther* 80: 997–1003, 2000.

49. Freitas SR, Mendes B, Le Sant G, Andrade RJ, Nordez A, and Milanovic Z. Can chronic stretching change the muscle-tendon mechanical properties? A review. *Scand J Med Sci Sports* 28 (3): 794–806, 2018.

50. da Silva JJ, Behm DG, Gomes WA, Silva FH, Soares EG, Serpa EP, Vilela Gde B, Jr, Lopes CR, and Marchetti PH. Unilateral plantar flexors static-stretching effects on ipsilateral and contralateral jump measures. *J Sports Sci Med* 14: 315–321, 2015.

51. Marchetti PH, Silva FH, Soares EG, Serpa EP, Nardi PS, Vilela Gde B, and Behm DG. Upper limb static-stretching protocol decreases maximal concentric jump performance. *J Sports Sci Med* 13: 945–950, 2014.

52. Marchetti PHR, Reis RG, Gomes WA, da Silva JJ, Soares EG, de Freitas FS, and Behm DG. Static-stretching of the pectoralis major decreases triceps brachii activation during a maximal isometric bench press. *Gazzetta Medica Italiana* 176 (12): 659–664, 2017.

53. Beighton P, Solomon L, and Soskolne CL. Articular mobility in an African population. *Ann Rheum Dis* 32: 413–418, 1973.

54. Biro F, Gewanter HL, and Baum J. The hypermobility syndrome. *Pediatrics* 72: 701–706, 1983.

55. Decoster LC, Vailas JC, Lindsay RH, and Williams GR. Prevalence and features of joint hypermobility among adolescent athletes. *Arch Pediatr Adolesc Med* 151: 989–992, 1997.

56. Larsson LG, Baum J, and Mudholkar GS. Hypermobility: features and differential incidence between the sexes. *Arthritis Rheum* 30: 1426–1430, 1987.

57. Wordsworth P, Ogilvie D, Smith R, and Sykes B. Joint mobility with particular reference to racial variation and inherited connective tissue disorders. *Br J Rheumatol* 26: 9–12, 1987.

58. Russek LN. Hypermobility syndrome. *Phys Ther* 79: 591–599, 1999.

59. Barrack RL, Skinner HB, Brunet ME, and Cook SD. Joint laxity and proprioception in the knee. *Phys Sportsmed* 11: 130–135, 1983.

60. Mallik AK, Ferrell WR, McDonald AG, and Sturrock RD. Impaired proprioceptive acuity at the proximal interphalangeal joint in patients with the hypermobility syndrome. *Br J Rheumatol* 33: 631–637, 1994.

61. Beighton PG, Grahame R, and Bird H. *Hypermobility of Joints*. London: Springer-Verlag, 1999.

62. Finsterbush A and Pogrund H. The hypermobility syndrome. Musculoskeletal complaints in 100 consecutive cases of generalized joint hypermobility. *Clin Orthop Relat Res* 168: 124–127, 1982.

63. Grahame R. Joint hypermobility – clinical aspects. *Proc R Soc Med* 64: 692–694, 1971.

64. Altman GH, Horan RL, Martin I, Farhadi J, Stark PR, Volloch V, Richmond JC, Vunjak-Novakovic G, and Kaplan DL. Cell differentiation by mechanical stress. *FASEB J* 16: 270–272, 2002.

65. Arnoczky SP, Lavagnino M, Egerbacher M, Caballero O, Gardner K, and Shender MA. Loss of homeostatic strain alters mechanostat "set point" of tendon cells in vitro. *Clin Orthop Relat Res* 466: 1583–1591, 2008.

66. Tyrance HJ. Relationships of extreme body types to ranges of flexibility. *Res Quart* 3: 349–359, 1958.

67. Sunderland S. *Traumatized Nerves, Roots and Ganglia. Musculoskeletal Factors and Neuropathological Consequences*. New York: Plenum Press, 1978.

68. Sunderland S. *Nerve Injuries and Their Repair. A Critical Appraisal.* London: Churchill Livingstone, 1991.
69. Grewal R, Xu J, Sotereanos DG, and Woo SL. Biomechanical properties of peripheral nerves. *Hand Clin* 12: 195–1204, 1996.
70. Lundborg G. Structure and function of the intraneural microvessels as related to trauma, edema formation, and nerve function. *J Bone Joint Surg Am* 57: 938–948, 1975.
71. Lundborg G and Rydevik B. Effects of stretching the tibial nerve of the rabbit. A preliminary study of the intraneural circulation and the barrier function of the perineurium. *J Bone Joint Surg Br* 55: 390–401, 1973.
72. Ogata K and Naito M. Blood flow of peripheral nerve effects of dissection, stretching and compression. *J Hand Surg Br* 11: 10–14, 1986.
73. Wall EJ, Massie JB, Kwan MK, Rydevik BL, Myers RR, and Garfin SR. Experimental stretch neuropathy. Changes in nerve conduction under tension. *J Bone Joint Surg Br* 74: 126–129, 1992.
74. Sunderland SB and Bradley KC. Stress-strain phenomena in human spinal nerve roots. *Brain* 84: 102–119, 1961.
75. Smith JW. Factors influencing nerve repair. I. Blood supply of peripheral nerves. *Arch Surg* 93: 335–341, 1966.
76. Leighton JR. Flexibility characteristics of males ten to eighteen years of age. *Arch Phys Med Rehabil* 37: 494–499, 1956.
77. Massey BAC and Chaudet NL. Effects of systematic, heavy resistance exercise on range of joint movements in young adults. *Res Quart* 27: 41–51, 1956.
78. Schmitt GDP, Pelham TW, and Holt LE. Changes in flexibility of elite female soccer players resulting from a flexibility program or combined flexibility and strength program: A pilot study. *Clin Kinesiol* 52: 64–67, 1998.
79. Wickstrom RL. Weight training and flexibility. *J Health Phys Educ Recreat* 34: 61–62, 1963.
80. Wilmore JH, Parr RB, Girandola RN, Ward P, Vodak PA, Barstow TJ, Pipes TV, Romero GT, and Leslie P. Physiological alterations consequent to circuit weight training. *Med Sci Sports* 10: 79–84, 1978.
81. Barbosa AR, Santarem JM, Filho WJ and Marucci Mde F. Effects of resistance training on the sit-and-reach test in elderly women. *J Strength Cond Res* 16: 14–18, 2002.
82. Fatouros IG, Taxildaris K, Tokmakidis SP, Kalapotharakos V, Aggelousis N, Athanasopoulos S, Zeeris I, and Katrabasas I. The effects of strength training, cardiovascular training and their combination on flexibility of inactive older adults. *Int J Sports Med* 23: 112–119, 2002.
83. Girouard CK and Hurley BF. Does strength training inhibit gains in range of motion from flexibility training in older adults? *Med Sci Sports Exerc* 27: 1444–1449, 1995.
84. Gao M, Sotomayor M, Villa E, Lee EH, and Schulten K. Molecular mechanisms of cellular mechanics. *Phys Chem Chem Phys* 8: 3692–3706, 2006.
85. Huang H, Kamm RD, and Lee RT. Cell mechanics and mechanotransduction: pathways, probes, and physiology. *Am J Physiol Cell Physiol* 287: C1–C11, 2004.
86. Zanchi NE and Lancha AH, Jr. Mechanical stimuli of skeletal muscle: Implications on mTOR/p70s6k and protein synthesis. *Eur J Appl Physiol* 102: 253–263, 2008.
87. Boppart MD, Burkin DJ, and Kaufman SJ. Alpha$_7$beta$_1$-integrin regulates mechanotransduction and prevents skeletal muscle injury. *Am J Physiol Cell Physiol* 290: C1660–C1665, 2006.

88. Laurent G and Sparrow M. Changes in RNA, DNA and protein content and the rates of protein synthesis and degradation during hypertrophy of the anterior latissimus dorsi muscle of the adult fowl (gallus domesticus). *Growth* 41: 249–262, 1977.

89. McHugh MP and Cosgrave CH. To stretch or not to stretch: the role of stretching in injury prevention and performance. *Scand J Med Sci Sports* 20: 169–181, 2010.

90. Nakamura M, Ikezoe T, Kobayashi T, Umegaki H, Takeno Y, Nishishita S, and Ichihashi N. Acute effects of static stretching on muscle hardness of the medial gastrocnemius muscle belly in humans: An ultrasonic shear-wave elastography study. *Ultrasound Med Biol* 40: 1991–1997, 2014.

91. Abellaneda S, Guissard N, and Duchateau J. The relative lengthening of the myotendinous structures in the medial gastrocnemius during passive stretching differs among individuals. *J Appl Physiol* 106: 169–177, 2009.

92. Magnusson SP, Narici MV, Maganaris CN, and Kjaer M. Human tendon behaviour and adaptation, in vivo. *J Physiol* 586: 71–81, 2008.

93. Blazevich AJ, Cannavan D, Waugh CM, Miller SC, Thorlund JB, Aagaard P, and Kay AD. Range of motion, neuromechanical, and architectural adaptations to plantar flexor stretch training in humans. *J Appl Physiol (1985)* 117: 452–462, 2014.

94. Nakamura M, Ikezoe T, Tokugawa T, and Ichihashi N. Acute effects of stretching on passive properties of human gastrocnemius muscle-tendon unit: Analysis of differences between hold-relax and static stretching. *J Sport Rehabil* 24: 286–292, 2015.

95. Azevedo DC, Melo RM, Alves Correa RV, and Chalmers G. Uninvolved versus target muscle contraction during contract:relax proprioceptive neuromuscular facilitation stretching. *Phys Ther Sport* 12: 117–121, 2011.

96. Etnyre BR and Lee EJ. Chronic and acute flexibility of men and women using 3 different stretching techniques. *Res Q Exercise Sport* 59: 222–228, 1988.

97. Ferber R, Osternig L, and Gravelle D. Effect of PNF stretch techniques on knee flexor muscle EMG activity in older adults. *J Electromyogr Kinesiol* 12: 391–397, 2002.

98. Freitas SR, Vilarinho D, Rocha Vaz J, Bruno PM, Costa PB, and Mil-Homens P. Responses to static stretching are dependent on stretch intensity and duration. *Clin Physiol Funct Imaging* 35: 478–484, 2015.

99. O'Hora J, Cartwright A, Wade CD, Hough AD, and Shum GL. Efficacy of static stretching and proprioceptive neuromuscular facilitation stretch on hamstrings length after a single session. *J Strength Cond Res/Natl Strength Cond Assoc* 25: 1586–1591, 2011.

100. Condon SM and Hutton RS. Soleus muscle electromyographic activity and ankle dorsiflexion range of motion during four stretching procedures. *Phys Ther* 67: 24–30, 1987.

101. Maddigan ME, Peach AA, and Behm DG. A comparison of assisted and unassisted proprioceptive neuromuscular facilitation techniques and static stretching. *J Strength Cond Res/Natl Strength Cond Assoc* 26: 1238–1244, 2012.

102. Borges MO, Medeiros DM, Minotto BB, and Lima CS. Comparison between static stretching and proprioceptive neuromuscular facilitation on hamstring flexibility: systematic review and meta-analysis. *Eur J Physiotherapy* 20 (1), 12–19, 2018.

103. Thomas E, Bianco A, Paoli A, and Palma A. The relation between stretching typology and stretching duration: the effects on range of motion. *Int J Sports Med* 39: 243–254, 2018.

104. Fletcher IM. The effect of different dynamic stretch velocities on jump performance. *Eur J Appl Physiol* 109: 491–498, 2010.

105. Mutungi G and Ranatunga KW. Temperature-dependent changes in the viscoelasticity of intact resting mammalian (rat) fast- and slow-twitch muscle fibres. *J Physiol* 508 (Pt 1): 253–265, 1998.

106. Herda TJ, Herda ND, Costa PB, Walter-Herda AA, Valdez AM, and Cramer JT. The effects of dynamic stretching on the passive properties of the muscle-tendon unit. *J Sports Sci* 31: 479–487, 2013.
107. Warren CG, Lehmann JF, and Koblanski JN. Elongation of rat tail tendon: Effect of load and temperature. *Arch Phys Med Rehabil* 52: 465–474 passim, 1971.
108. Warren CG, Lehmann JF, and Koblanski JN. Heat and stretch procedures: An evaluation using rat tail tendon. *Arch Phys Med Rehabil* 57: 122–126, 1976.
109. Taylor DC, Dalton JD, Jr., Seaber AV, and Garrett WE, Jr. Viscoelastic properties of muscle-tendon units. The biomechanical effects of stretching. *Am J Sports Med* 18: 300–309, 1990.

5

TRAINING-RELATED RANGE OF MOTION CHANGES AND MECHANISMS

Chronic stretching (training) can increase range of motion (ROM) using different stretching techniques, positions, and durations (1). Naturally, there are always dissenting findings as, for example: 4 (10 repetitions of 30 s, 3 days/week) (2) or 6 (4 repetitions of 45 s, 4 days/week) (3) weeks of hamstrings static stretching did not increase hip extension or flexion ROM, respectively. But the vast majority of stretch-training programmes do exhibit ROM improvements (4–8). But which type of stretch training is most effective? A review by Decoster et al. (1) indicated that static stretch training provided greater ROM improvements than PNF. Other studies have documented static stretch-induced ROM improvements with no improvements with PNF (30-second stretch, 3 days/week for 4 weeks) (5), whereas another study found training-induced ROM improvements with no difference between static and PNF stretching (4 days/week for 6 weeks) (8). Although one study reported more than double the ROM improvements with static stretching versus dynamic stretching (9), others have not shown any significant difference (10). Hence, it seems that the literature cannot provide a definitive answer about the most effective form of stretch training for plastic (semi-permanent) ROM increases, albeit all stretching programmes consistently provide significant training-related improvements.

The persistence of these flexibility adaptations after stretch training desists have been reported to show better than pre-training ROM for 3 (11), 4 (12, 13), and 8 (14) weeks. Similar to strength training, a maintenance flexibility training programme of one session per week can help preserve the training gains (15). Similar to elastic (acute) ROM responses, plastic ROM changes or changes attributed to flexibility training can also be attributed to a variety of factors, including neural, morphological, and psychological. Which of these factors is most predominant is still under debate.

Plastic neural adaptations

Is it possible that the neural inhibitory responses that occur with elastic or acute changes in ROM can persist or be semi-permanent with training or plastic changes? Just as with the neural adaptations associated with strength training, prolonged alterations in the nervous system can evolve with flexibility training. Blazevich et al. (16) incorporated a 3-week stretch-training programme of the plantar flexors and found a reduction in tonic Ia (facilitatory) afferent feedback from muscle spindles (measured from the tendon or T-reflex). So, when the spindles were stretched, their firing frequency was less than before the flexibility training, resulting in less reflex-induced contractions and a more relaxed muscle (disfacilitation). Perhaps the decreased spindle activity was due to increased compliance (reduced stiffness) of the passive elastic components. Thus, with a certain degree of stretch, the tissues around the spindles would accommodate the elongation, and the spindle would not be stretched or elongated to the same extent resulting in a muted reflex response. However, in their study, the T-reflex reduction (spindle activity) did not parallel the reduction in passive stiffness during the stretch-training programme. Therefore, if the reduced spindle activity cannot be attributed to lower tissue compliance, then it is more likely that the flexibility training led to an intrinsic reduction in muscle spindle sensitivity. In this case, the stretch training had a direct effect on the activity of the nervous system (afferent input to the motoneurons). In the same Blazevich study, they also reported increased reciprocal inhibition in soleus and gastrocnemius, which would decrease the contractile force of the antagonists. Guissard and Duchateau had participants stretch 5 days/week for 6 weeks (4 stretch positions × 5 repetitions × 30 seconds each) and tested immediately after the training programme, as well as after 1 month of detraining. Similar to the Blazevich et al. findings, they also found decreases in Hoffmann or H- and T-reflexes (−36% and −14%, respectively). However, they found that the reflex inhibition was present after the first 10 stretching sessions, but returned to baseline when tested after 30 days of detraining. On the other hand, passive muscle stiffness was apparent at every point from 10 days of training to 30 days of detraining (17).

Plastic morphological adaptations

Stretch-training studies in animal models have demonstrated sarcomerogenesis (increased number of sarcomeres in series) (18), but there is very limited or no evidence in humans. However, once again it should be pointed out that there are no longitudinal studies examining stretch-induced morphological changes over years of stretching. Again, with animal studies, stretch is a very potent signal for mechano-growth factor (MGF: a variant of insulin growth factor 1 or IGF-1), actin and myosin filament production, myosin isoform gene switching, protein turnover, and hypertrophy, as well as for adding sarcomeres in parallel and series (19–22).

Traditionally, PNF stretching effects were attributed primarily to neural inhibition (e.g. reciprocal inhibition, autogenic inhibition). However, there is a lack of experimental evidence for this emphasis on neural responses (23, 24). The effectiveness of PNF may be due to an increased tolerance to stretch (25) but there can also be morphological changes. For example, 6 weeks of PNF flexibility training reduced the passive and active stiffness of the Achilles tendon while also increasing the pennation angle of gastrocnemius. However, there was no change in the passive–resistive torque of the muscle (26). Significant reductions in the myotendinous junction (muscle and tendon intersection) stiffness (e.g. 47%) during a passive static stretch have also been reported after stretch training (27), and this decreased passive stiffness can contribute to increased flexibility (17). On the contrary, a 6-week (5 days/week) static stretch-training programme improved hip flexion ROM but did not change muscle extensibility (4). The authors therefore attributed the improved ROM to increased stretch tolerance. Static stretch training (2 days/week for 20 days) has been reported to reduce the tendon viscoelastic properties but not the tendon stiffness (28). Static stretch training (7 days/week for 6 weeks) improved dorsiflexion ROM with a reduced muscle passive resistive torque, but no change in tendon stiffness, whereas ballistic stretch training exhibited the opposite effect with no change in muscle passive–resistive torque but decreased tendon stiffness (6). A review on chronic stretching changes reported that stretch training durations of 3–8 weeks (average study 5.1 weeks) do not alter muscle or tendon properties, although it can increase the extensibility and tolerance of the muscle to a greater tensile force (29). They also reported that these durations of stretching also have trivial effects on tendon properties. Although their review supports the stretch tolerance theory, you have to ask yourself if most athletes or fitness enthusiasts stretch for only 5 weeks or less than 2 months. Many athletes will have stretched on a regular basis from adolescence to early adulthood and may continue on a less vigorous or consistent basis for many years hence. Thus, examining studies of only a maximum of 8 weeks' duration does not provide a full picture of possible chronic morphological changes.

It would be fantastic for the public if the studies found consistent results, but each study may use different types of stretching, durations, volumes, intensities, and subject populations. The most prudent comment or recommendation might be to incorporate a variety of stretching styles (static, dynamic, and PNF) in order to ensure that morphological changes to the muscle and tendons is optimized by providing a variety of stressors to the system.

Psychological adaptations

Although the training-induced increase in joint ROM can be connected to neural and morphological alterations, there is also a strong case for an increase in stretch tolerance (25, 30). This is also known as the sensory theory, which indicates the musculotendinous unit can tolerate greater tensions without a change in tension for a given length; 60 individuals stretched for 30 minutes, 5 times/week for 6 weeks with no change in hamstring extensibility. As there was an increase in the ROM, the authors suggest that the improvement must have been due to greater stretch tolerance (4).

Summary

Although there is still conflict in the literature, generally static and PNF stretching tend to provide greater improvements with static ROM than dynamic stretching. Flexibility training adaptations can persist for 3–8 weeks with either reduced (once a week) or minimal stretching and activity. This persistent flexibility adaptations may be partially ascribed to neural adaptations such as an intrinsic disfacilitation of spindle afferent discharge. Although animal stretching studies have shown an increase in sarcomeres in series, there are no similar human findings with flexibility training. However, there is evidence with human chronic flexibility training for alterations in muscle pennation angles, viscoelastic properties, and stretch tolerance.

References

1. Decoster LC, Cleland J, Altieri C, and Russell P. The effects of hamstring stretching on range of motion: A systematic literature review. *J Orthop Sports Phys Ther* 35: 377–387, 2005.
2. LaRoche DP, Lussier MV, and Roy SJ. Chronic stretching and voluntary muscle force. *J Strength Cond Res* 22: 589–596, 2008.
3. Bazett-Jones DM, Gibson MH, and McBride JM. Sprint and vertical jump performances are not affected by six weeks of static hamstring stretching. *J Strength Cond Res* 22: 25–31, 2008.
4. Ben M and Harvey LA. Regular stretch does not increase muscle extensibility: a randomized controlled trial. *Scand J Med Sci Sports*, 2009.
5. Davis DS, Ashby PE, McHale KL, McQuain JA, and Wine JM. The effectiveness of 3 stretching techniques on hamstring flexibility using consistent stretching parameters. *J Strength Cond Res* 19: 27–32, 2005.
6. Mahieu NN, McNair P, De Muynck M, Stevens V, Blanckaert I, Smits N, and Witvrouw E. Effect of static and ballistic stretching on the muscle-tendon tissue properties. *Med Sci Sports Exerc* 39: 494–501, 2007.
7. Nelson AG, Kokkonen J, Eldredge C, Cornwell A, and Glickman-Weiss E. Chronic stretching and running economy. *Scand J Med Sci Sports* 11: 260–265, 2001.
8. Yuktasir B and Kaya F. Investigation into the long term effects of static and PNF stretching exercises on range of motion and jump preformance. *J Bodyw Mov Ther* 13: 11–21, 2009.
9. Bandy WD, Irion JM, and Briggler M. The effect of static stretch and dynamic range of motion training on the flexibility of the hamstring muscles. *J Orthop Sports Phys Ther* 27: 295–300, 1998.
10. Wiemann K and Hahn K. Influences of strength, stretching and circulatory exercises on flexibility parameters of the human hamstrings. *Int J Sports Med* 18: 340–346, 1997.
11. Long PA. *The effect of static, dynamic, and combined stretching exercise programs on the hip joint flexibility*. Baltimore, MA: University of Maryland, 1971.

12. Tweitmeyer TA. A comparison of two stretching techniques for increasing and retaining flexibility. Iowa City, IA: University of Iowa Press, 1974.
13. Zebas CJ and Rivera ML. Retention of flexibility in selected joints after cessation of a stretching exercise program. In: *Exercise physiology current selected research I*. New York AMS Press, 1985, pp 181–191.
14. McCue BF. Flexibility measurement of college women. *Res Q* 3: 316–324, 1963.
15. Wallin D, Ekblom B, Grahn R, and Nordenberg T. Improvement of muscle flexibility: a comparison between two techniques. *Am J Sport Med* 13: 263–267, 1985.
16. Blazevich AJ, Cannavan D, Waugh CM, Fath F, Miller SC, and Kay AD. Neuromuscular factors influencing the maximum stretch limit of the human plantar flexors. *J Appl Physiol* 113: 1446–1455, 2012.
17. Guissard N and Duchateau J. Effect of static stretch training on neural and mechanical properties of the human plantar-flexor muscles. *Muscle Nerve* 29: 248–255, 2004.
18. De Jaeger D, Joumaa V, and Herzog W. Intermittent stretch training of rabbit plantar-flexor muscles increases soleus mass and serial sarcomere number. *J Appl Physiol (1985)* 118: 1467–1473, 2015.
19. Goldspink D. The influence of passive stretch on the growth and protein turnover of the denervated extensor digitorum longus muscle. *Biochem J* 174: 595–602, 1978.
20. Goldspink DF. The influence of immobilization and stretch on protein turnover of rat skeletal muscle. *J Physiol* 264: 267–282, 1977.
21. Goldspink G. Changes in muscle mass and phenotype and the expression of autocrine and systemic growth factors by muscle in response to stretch and overload. *J Anat* 194 (Pt 3): 323–334, 1999.
22. Goldspink G, Scutt A, Martindale J, Jaenicke T, Gerlach G, and Turay L. Stretch and force generation induce rapid hypertrophy and myosin isoform gene switching in adult skeletal muscle. *Biochem Soc Trans* 19: 368–373, 1990.
23. Chalmers G. Re-examination of the possible role of Golgi tendon organ and muscle spindle reflexes in proprioceptive neuromuscular facilitation muscle stretching. *Sports Biomech* 3: 159–183, 2004.
24. Sharman MJ, Cresswell AG, and Riek S. Proprioceptive neuromuscular facilitation stretching: mechanisms and clinical implications. *Sports Med* 36: 929–939, 2006.
25. Magnusson SP, Simonsen EB, Aagaard P, Sorensen H, and Kjaer M. A mechanism for altered flexibility in human skeletal muscle. *J Physiol* 497 (Pt 1): 291–298, 1996.
26. Konrad A, Gad M, and Tilp M. Effect of PNF stretching training on the properties of human muscle and tendon structures. *Scand J Med Sci Sports* 25: 346–355, 2015.
27. Morse CI, Degens H, Seynnes OR, Maganaris CN, and Jones DA. The acute effect of stretching on the passive stiffness of the human gastrocnemius muscle tendon unit. *J Physiol* 586: 97–106, 2008.
28. Kubo K, Kanehisa H, and Fukunaga T. Effect of stretching training on the viscoelastic properties of human tendon structures in vivo. *J Appl Physiol* 92: 595–601, 2002.
29. Freitas SR, Mendes B, Le Sant G, Andrade RJ, Nordez A, and Milanovic Z. Can chronic stretching change the muscle-tendon mechanical properties? a review. *Scand J Med Sci Sports* 22 September, 2017.
30. Magnusson P and Renstrom P. The European College of Sports Sciences Position statement: the role of stretching exercises in sports. *Eur J Sport Sci* 6: 87–91, 2006.

6

RECOMMENDATIONS FOR STRETCHING PRESCRIPTION

Stretching duration

Almost any duration of stretching can improve range of motion (ROM). In almost every study, you read, the very act of measuring a joint ROM will improve elastic flexibility. In one of our studies we found we needed to pre-test individuals at least three times to ensure that the ROM did not increase due just to the testing (1). Thus, a single stretch of ≤5 seconds may improve ROM (2). This is why every stretching study needs a control condition or group! Whereas Roberts and Wilson (2) showed that nine stretches of 5 seconds provided similar increases in passive ROM as three stretches of 15 seconds, the 15-second stretches had a significantly better effect on active ROM than the 5-second stretches. Earlier studies by Bandy and Irion (3) suggested that 30–60 seconds of static stretching was more effective than 15 seconds to increase passive ROM. A static stretch training study had participants train three times a week for 5 weeks and found significant improvements in ROM with 5-second stretch training but 15 seconds of stretching provided greater improvements (2). Other researchers also support using more than 30 seconds of static stretching to achieve the greatest ROM (4,5). In a later study by Bandy et al. (6) they indicated that one 30-second static stretch per day increased hamstring ROM, but there were no differences with increased repetitions or frequency. In an animal study using rabbits (7) it was found that the greatest length changes in the musculotendinous unit (MTU) occurred within the first four stretches. In humans, two 30-second static stretches were needed to decrease musculotendinous stiffness of the plantar flexors significantly (8). There were no further decreases with three to four stretches of the same duration. Although we are obviously not the same as rabbits, the findings with these warm-blooded mammalian cousins, in association with some of the human studies, tend to provide the same message: there is no need for an exaggerated duration of stretching to obtain acute optimal increases in ROM. Thomas et al. (9), in their meta-analysis, recommended a minimum duration of 5 min/week for each muscle group.

Stretching intensity

Many studies utilize static stretches that elongate the MTU or joint to the point of discomfort (pain) or near the point of discomfort (10–14). Mechanically, this stretch point would be referred to as the elastic limit, which is the minimum amount of stress placed on a tissue to elicit permanent strain. Exceeding the elastic limit will result in the tissue not returning to its original length after the stretch (15). At this point, musculotendinous strains or ligamentous sprain injuries could occur. Alter (15) expands on the strength-training overload principle (16–18), transferring the concept to flexibility training as the overstretching principle, which is described as "when the body is regularly stimulated by an increasingly intense stretching program beyond the homeostatic level, it will respond with an increased ability to stretch" (15, p. 145). The question arises of whether it is necessary to reach the elastic limit or point of discomfort to achieve plastic or semi-permanent changes in flexibility.

A number of acute studies have shown that submaximal intensity stretches provide similar ROM benefits to stretches that are near to the maximal point of discomfort (19–22). We had participants stretch at 100%, 75%, and 50% of the point of discomfort, but found no significant difference in the flexibility test (stoop and reach). All conditions improved by approximately 12% (13). In contrast, another study reported that static stretching at 85–100% of maximum stretch intensity provided greater ROM than stretching at 60% (23). Other studies have compared high force–short duration with low force–long duration stretching, and report that high-force stretches emphasize elastic tissue deformation which shortly returns to its original length, whereas low-force, prolonged stretching enhances plastic or semi-permanent changes in tissue length (24–27). Apostopoulos (28) recommended stretching at 30–40% of perceived exertion. Stretching to the point of pain could be counterproductive. A typical response to pain, discomfort, or distress is to adopt a stiffening strategy (29), i.e. to contract both the agonist and antagonist muscles in order to protect them from possible physical insults. Hence, while the individual is trying to lengthen the muscle, the central nervous system is trying to shorten the muscle. So, there is no need for masochism when stretching; pain is not a necessity. Furthermore, stretching to the point of discomfort or elastic limit for a recently injured or fatigued tissue could strain (muscles and tendons) or sprain (ligaments) the tissue. Thus, during rehabilitation or after an intense, fatiguing, training session or match, high-intensity stretching should not be pursued. Another point to consider is that pain is highly subjective to the individual. Hence, telling a person with a high pain threshold to stretch to the point of discomfort will place much greater stress on the tissues than for someone who has a lower tolerance to pain. It is much safer and reportedly equally effective to stretch below pain tolerance!

Continuous stretching (no rest periods) permits higher stretching intensities (30). However, as mentioned earlier, higher stretching intensities may not provide any extra ROM benefits. In fact, one study reported that intermittent stretching reduced peak torque (i.e. strength) more than continuous stretching, which was strongly associated with a depression in central drive (31).

Optimal time of day to stretch

When is the best time of day to stretch? There are diurnal (time-of-day) variations in performance. Typically, most people perform maximal strength and power activities better in the afternoon compared with the morning. Dynamic stretching has been shown to counteract the lower vertical jump heights often found in the morning (32). Dr Stuart McGill, a highly respected biomechanist (with one of the best moustaches around), from the University of Waterloo, suggests that extensive stretching in the morning is counterproductive. Vertebral discs are infused with fluid known as the nucleus pulposa. After a night of being horizontal during sleep, the disc's nucleus pulposa becomes more hydrated. The gravity-induced fluid loss due to a day of upright posture is replaced. This modulation in fluid alters the stresses on the disc throughout the day. Specifically, stress is highest after bed rest and then diminishes over the subsequent few hours. Stretching the lower back in the morning with the discs expanded can increase the chances of disc herniation. Passive tissues of the back can be injured by bending over to pick up a pencil, especially if the individual is unstable. Thus, attempting to touch the toes whether in the morning or any other time of the day can lead to injury. In fact, McGill proposes that a more flexible back actually increases the risk of future back problems. He states there is trade-off between mobility and stability, and that balance is specific to the individual based on previous injuries, age, training objectives, and other factors (33).

Stretching frequency (days/week)

Should we stretch every day or alternate days? To my knowledge, there are very few to no studies that have directly compared the frequency of stretch training. Perhaps examination of the strength-training literature would be helpful on this issue. Resistance training the same muscle on subsequent days is not advised because the muscle needs time to recover. If the intensity is sufficient, overload resistance stress can degrade muscle protein and activate a number of receptors and pathways for increased protein synthesis. This overcompensation to the stress can result in increased muscle strength and hypertrophy (34–36). However, without a sufficient recovery period (typically 48–72 hours), the muscle pathways continue to emphasize protein degradation rather than the synthesis of protein, resulting in decreased strength and atrophy. For the most extreme example, contemplate the muscle hypertrophy of a bodybuilder against the muscle atrophy of a war-time concentration camp prisoner. Both individuals receive an overload stress on the muscle, but the bodybuilder builds appropriate rest periods (and of course proper nutrition) into the programme whereas the prisoner works hard every day without the chance for overcompensation. The difference between resistance training and stretching is the lower overload intensity and lack of protein degradation with stretching. Most stretching programmes would not lead to similar protein degradation or depletion of muscle glycogen stores as resistance training, and thus there would not be a need for a prolonged recovery period. There is ample evidence of individuals who stretch every day providing significant improvements in flexibility without any negative consequences. It is possible that extreme flexibility programmes, as seen with some gymnasts, dancers, and other similar athletes, may damage muscle and connective tissue and might be more effective with alternate-day stretching. However, this type of comparative research has not been conducted. Flexibility training studies have successfully improved ROM with flexibility training programmes of 2 (37), 3 (38), 4 (39), 5 (40), and 7 (41–45) days/week. As can be seen from the number of citations, daily stretching has been commonly used in the literature. Thus, for the vast majority of people who stretch, daily stretching should provide substantial improvements in flexibility. As mentioned previously, stretching only 1 day/ week can sustain previously attained flexibility training gains (46). As no extensive direct comparison studies (i.e. one study that directly compared 1 vs 3 vs 5 vs 7 days of stretching per week) have been conducted, we cannot state whether daily stretching actually provides better flexibility improvements than 5 days/week, 3 days/week, or other frequencies. However, the meta-analysis of Thomas et al. (9), comparing the results of studies using differing stretching frequencies, suggested that stretching at least 5 days per week (with a minimum 5 min per muscle group per week) provided the most beneficial increases in ROM. Furthermore, although Alter (15) suggests that stretching once a day would maintain flexibility and "empirical evidence suggests that stretching at least twice a day is preferable" (p. 154), there is scant evidence about whether stretching multiple times per day substantially enhances the improvement in flexibility. We plan on investigating these questions soon in our lab.

Pre- versus post-workout stretching

Should we stretch before or after a workout? Chapter 8 deals with the effects of pre-activity stretching during a warm-up, so we leave that discussion till then. A common practice is to perform stretching exercises after a workout, with the rationale being that the muscles and connective tissue are warm and the viscosity is low. This decreased viscosity is certainly an advantage for achieving greater muscle and tendon lengths, but dependent on previous activity, the muscles may be fatigued as well. Hence, attempting to stretch musculotendinous tissue to the maximum point of discomfort in order to achieve greater extensibility could lead to tissue strains if the tensile strength of the tissue is compromised by fatigue. Therefore, post-exercise stretching, especially if fatigue is induced, should involve low-to-moderate intensity stretching, so as not to overload the tension on the muscles and tendons. This stretching period should be more in the relaxation mode than to increase musculotendinous extensibility!

Stretching for relaxation

Static stretching can physiologically relax an individual. Static stretching (5 repetitions × 1 minute each of triceps surae) changed the predominance of the autonomic nervous system to a greater parasympathetic neural influence during the stretch and continued for 4 minutes after the stretch (47). This effect can last substantially longer because another study found the greater parasympathetic influence returning to pre-stretch levels 30 minutes after stretching (3 stretches × 30 seconds each) (48). Relaxation can be an important aspect of exercise recovery. High stress, whether physiological or psychological, can increases cortisol (49). Cortisol, a catabolic hormone, increases protein degradation, increases the metabolism of protein, fat, and carbohydrates, and suppresses the immune system (50). With recovery, we basically want the opposite actions to occur. Thus, although high-intensity stretching is not recommended after a workout with the objective of increasing ROM, stretching in order to relax would be a strong recommendation after taxing physical activity.

In addition to stretching, a focus on breathing patterns can affect parasympathetic activation. Yoga, of course, has developed and focused on a variety of ventilatory strategies for centuries.

Ventilatory effects on stretching

A growing body of evidence supports the belief that yoga benefits physical and mental health via down-regulation of the hypothalamic–pituitary–adrenal (HPA) axis and the sympathetic nervous system (51). With yoga, the emphasis is often on deep, rhythmic, consistent, diaphragmatic, and nasal breathing to relax the individual (52). In a more relaxed state, it is believed that the individual will be able to achieve greater ROM. Unpublished data from our lab showed that unilateral nasal breathing could affect heart rate. While walking on a treadmill for 10 minutes, with unilateral left nostril breathing, there were significant increases in heart rate, and systolic and diastolic blood pressures. Post-treadmill walking, flexibility was tested and a significant decrease was found. In contrast, greater flexibility was achieved with decreased heart rate and blood pressure during walking after unilateral right nasal breathing. These results correspond with Yoga Tradition. Energy flow through "ida" (during left nasal breathing practice) is supposed to be "heat dissipating (cooling)", whereas energy flow through "pingala" (during right nasal breathing practice) is "heat generating". Hence, there may be a nostril laterality affecting the autonomous nervous system differentially (53), with left nostril breathing emphasizing the parasympathetic influence.

Similar to breathing or ventilatory patterns when resistance training, the breathing pattern can have an effect on stretching. especially when performing a trunk-forward flexion action. Expiring during trunk-forward flexion is typically recommended because a full inspiration tends to contract the erector spinae muscles (54,55) and expand the thoracic cage (ribs), which would detract from attempting to fully flex (15). In contrast, Hamilton and colleagues (56) found greater ROM and lower electromyographic (EMG) activity of rectus abdominis, external obliques, lower abdominal stabilizers, and lower erector spinae of women with breathing techniques that emphasized larger inhalations. There was no effect of different breathing techniques on the male participants. The greater joint stiffness of men (57) may have contributed to a lack of ventilatory effects. McHugh et al. (58) reported that mechanical factors contribute about 80% to the trunk-forward flexion ROM, and thus the intrinsic male mechanical stiffness may have overcome neural or mechanical ventilatory effects. For both sexes in the study, EMG activity while inhaling before the stretch was not significantly lower, which tends to indicate that relaxed trunk muscle activity is not the single most important factor for attaining greater flexibility, contradicting some earlier studies (54,55). Furthermore, pulmonary stretch reflexes inhibit sympathetic nerve activity at higher lung tidal volumes (59), thus there could have been lower sympathetic nerve activity for the pre-stretch inhale, inhale during stretch, and hypoventi- lation conditions in the Hamilton study. Hamilton recommended that women should inhale at a slow frequency (hypoventilation) before and maintain that inhalation during the stretch. In contrast to the earlier studies cited above, they found that forceful exhalations actually increased EMG activity, thus inhibiting hip flexion ROM.

Combining stretching with muscular contractions or massage

Other techniques might be applied during a stretch to augment ROM increases. Implementing muscular contractions during a static stretch (active static stretch) might provide some greater benefit early in a training programme (i.e. 4 weeks), but no additional benefit over a longer time period compared with passive stretching (i.e. 8 weeks) (60). Another technique that can augment the stretching effect is massage of the tendon. In a study from our laboratory (61), friction massage was applied to the hamstrings tendon for either 10 or 30 seconds before testing for hip flexion (hamstrings) ROM. Both durations provided 6–7% increase in ROM. The heat-induced friction of the massage would have decreased viscoelasticity and perhaps activated cutaneous and myofascial afferents, helping to inhibit reflex-induced contractions. Massaging the tendon either before or during the stretch can augment the effectiveness.

Effect of temperature on stretching

Another consideration would be to ensure the tissues are at a higher temperature (hyperthermia) when stretching. Increased tissue temperatures decrease tissue stiffness and increase extensibility (24,62,63). Tendon temperatures over 39.4°C (103°F) can augment plastic elongation (24,64), whereas tissue temperatures over 40°C (104°F) can enhance the viscous stress relaxation for collagen protein, also leading to greater plastic deformation (63,65,66). There are conflicting studies about hyperthermic applications, with increased ROM found after hot baths (67), hot packs (10 minutes) (68), ultrasound (69), and diathermy (70). However, a lack of ROM augmentation has been reported after applying moist heat (71) or an electric heating pad (20 minutes at 43°C) (72).

There is controversy over whether a hypothermic (cold) stretch provides the best tissue lengthening (68,73), or whether the hypothermic elongated position should be maintained until the tissue cools (e.g. application of ice) (74,75). Cryotherapy (application of cold) together with static (76) and PNF (77) stretching has demonstrated improved flexibility compared with stretching alone. Cryotherapy can induce anaesthetic effects, which would allow the individual to push past their usual point of discomfort and stretch farther (increased stretch tolerance). However, as with almost every scientific question, there are dissenting findings (78–80). For example, there were no significant improvements in ROM with the application of 10 minutes of cold water immersion (81) or ice packs (68). Although hypothermic applications (cryotherapy) can aid in pain tolerance, it would also lead to vasoconstriction (81) and increase tissue viscoelasticity (75). Sapega et al. (75) suggests that cold should be used for therapeutic conditions when the objective is to disrupt adhesions or there is substantial muscle spasticity.

Stretching under metastable conditions

There are some innovative stretch coaches who have combined stretching routines under relatively unstable conditions. For example, Mario Di Santo of Argentina (former national gymnastics champion) has gymnasts place one foot on the floor with another foot suspended from a Theraband (elastic band) attached to the ceiling. The athlete must stretch their muscles while maintaining stability and balance. A possible advantage of this type of active static stretching is the task specificity (82). Whereas many stretching routines are performed under passive (no active voluntary muscle contraction) conditions, it is difficult to conceive of many sports that do not involve voluntary contractions and the necessity to maintain a high degree of balance or to be in a state of strong metastability (83). Athletes and all individuals involved in activities of daily living continually move from states of stability (i.e. standing) to instability (movements such as walking and running) and return to stability again (i.e. return to the stance phase of walking or running). So, with a metastable state, an individual will move from a stable to a transiently unstable state (i.e. gymnast, figure skater, or skier leaves the ground/floor to perform a jump or flip or other manoeuvre) and then returns to their stable condition again. In many of these manoeuvres, a high degree of flexibility is necessary and the athlete is certainly not in a passive state. Stretching using unstable devices to create a metastable condition, accentuate task, or action or sport specificity, by placing the MTU in a lengthened state under active metastable conditions. Thus, it is not only a stretch workout but a technique and motor control session as well (Figure 6.1).

Summary

In summary, whereas single static stretches of 5 seconds can improve ROM, it is generally recommended that longer durations of 30–60 seconds provide optimal improvements in flexibility. It is not necessary to perform these stretches to the point of discomfort (100% intensity). Although some studies have shown improvements even when stretching at 30–40% of maximal intensity, it seems that a stretching intensity of 60–85% would provide the greatest benefits. There are diurnal variations with flexibility and stretching mid- to later in the day, when the body is warmer, decreasing viscoelasticity and possibly enhancing ROM. It is not recommended to stretch your back early in the morning when there is increased vertebral disc fluid pressure which could lead to disc protrusion injuries or nerve entrapment. There is no strong evidence for an optimal stretching

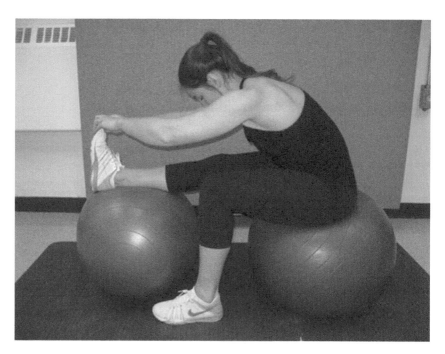

FIGURE 6.1 Stretching under unstable conditions to improve ROM and metastability

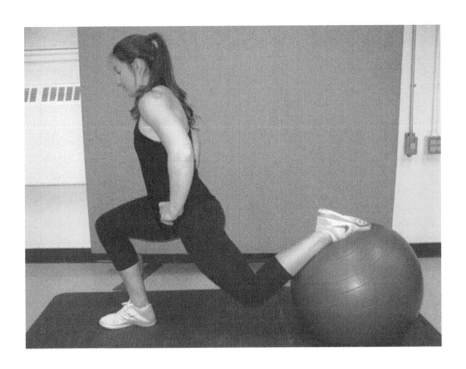

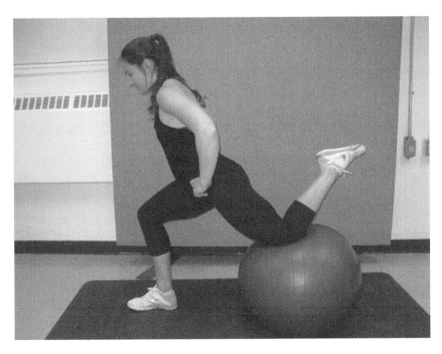

FIGURE 6.1 (Cont.)

frequency. However, as stretching is typically lower in intensity than resistance and high-intensity anaerobic training without significant protein catabolism or tissue damage, it can be practised every day, although significant increases in flexibility are also experienced when stretching 2 or 3–6 days/week. Whereas pre-event prolonged static stretching is not recommended due to the possibility of performance impairments, short-to-moderate duration static stretching (<60 seconds per muscle group) within a full warm-up, including dynamic stretching and dynamic activity, does not impair performance (see Chapter 8). Post-activity stretching might involve a fatigued MTU which could be susceptible to injury if subjected to intense elongation. Thus, post-activity stretching should be lower intensity, which can promote not only improvements in ROM but also psychological feelings of relaxation. When stretching, breathing patterns should be at a slow and controlled rate with a full tidal volume (large breaths) to promote greater relaxation. The breath should be expired or held as you approach the end of the ROM. Although stretching a warm muscle decreases viscoelasticity, promoting a greater ease of ROM, the use of cryotherapy, especially with intense stretching or rehabilitation, may increase stretch (pain) tolerance allowing the individual to push farther than normal.

References

1. Grabow L, Young JD, Alcock LR, Quigley PJ, Byrne JM, Granacher U, Skrabot J, and Behm DG. Higher quadriceps roller massage forces do not amplify range-of-motion increases or impair strength and jump performance. *J Strength Cond Res* doi:10.1519/JSC.0000000000001906, 2018.
2. Roberts JM and Wilson K. Effect of stretching duration on active and passive range of motion in the lower extremity. *Br J Sports Med* 33: 259–263, 1999.
3. Bandy WD and Irion JM. The effect of time on the static stretch of the hamstrings muscles. *Phys Ther* 74: 845–850, 1994.
4. Chan SP, Hong Y, and Robinson PD. Flexibility and passive resistance of the hamstrings of young adults using two different static stretching protocols. *Scand J Med Sci* 11: 81–86, 2001.
5. Feland JB, Myrer JW, Schulthies SS, Fellingham GW, and Measom GW. The effect of duration of stretching of the hamstring muscle group for increasing range of motion in people aged 65 years or older. *Phys Ther* 81: 1110–1117, 2001.
6. Bandy WD, Irion JM, and Briggler M. The effect of time and frequency of static stretching on flexibility of the hamstring muscles. *Phys Ther* 77: 1090–1096, 1997.
7. Taylor DC, Dalton JD, Seaber AV, and Garret WE. Viscoelastic properties of muscle-tendon units: the biomechanical effects of stretching. *Am J Sport Med* 18: 300–308, 1990.
8. Ryan ED, Herda TJ, Costa PB, Defreitas JM, Beck TW, Stout J, and Cramer JT. Determining the minimum number of passive stretches necessary to alter musculotendinous stiffness. *J Sports Sci* 27: 957–961, 2009.
9. Thomas E, Bianco A, Paoli A, and Palma A. The relation between stretching typology and stretching duration: the effects on range of motion. *Int J Sports Med* 39: 243–254, 2018.

10. Behm DG, Bambury A, Cahill F, and Power K. Effect of acute static stretching on force, balance, reaction time, and movement time. *Med Sci Sports Exerc* 36: 1397–1402, 2004.

11. Behm DG, Bradbury EE, Haynes AT, Hodder JN, Leonard AM, and Paddock NR. Flexibility is not related to stretch-induced deficits in force or power. *J Sports Sci Med* 5: 33–42, 2006.

12. Behm DG, Button DC, and Butt JC. Factors affecting force loss with prolonged stretching. *Can J Appl Physiol* 26: 261–272, 2001.

13. Behm DG and Kibele A. Effects of differing intensities of static stretching on jump performance. *Eur J Appl Physiol* 101: 587–594, 2007.

14. Behm DG, Plewe S, Grage P, Rabbani A, Beigi HT, Byrne JM, and Button DC. Relative static stretch-induced impairments and dynamic stretch-induced enhancements are similar in young and middle-aged men. *Appl Physiol Nutr Metab* 36: 790–797, 2011.

15. Alter MJ. *Science of flexibility*. Champaign Illinois: Human Kinetics, 1996.

16. Fleck S and Kraemer W. Resistance training: physiological responses and adaptations (Part 2 of 4). *Phys Sportsmed* 16: 108–118, 1988.

17. Fleck SJ and Kraemar WJ. Resistance training: Physiological responses and adaptations (Part 3 of 4). *Phys SportsMed* 16: 63–72, 1988.

18. Fleck SJ and Kraemer WJ. Resistance training: Basic principles (Part 1 of 4). *Phys SportsMed* 16: 108–114, 1988.

19. Knudson D, Bennett K, Corn R, Leick D, and Smith C. Acute effects of stretching are not evident in the kinematics of the vertical jump. *J Strength Cond Res* 15: 98–101, 2001.

20. Knudson DV, Noffal GJ, Bahamonde RE, Bauer JA, and Blackwell JR. Stretching has no effect on tennis serve performance. *J Strength Cond Res* 18: 654–656, 2004.

21. Manoel ME, Harris-Love MO, Danoff JV, and Miller TA. Acute effects of static, dynamic, and proprioceptive neuromuscular facilitation stretching on muscle power in women. *J Strength Cond Res* 22: 1528–1534, 2008.

22. Young W, Elias G, and Power J. Effects of static stretching volume and intensity on plantar flexor explosive force production and range of motion. *J Sports Med Phys Fitness* 46: 403–411, 2006.

23. Walter J, Figoni SF, Andres FF, and Brown E. Training intensity and duration in flexibility. *Clin Kinesiol* 2: 40–45, 1996.

24. Laban MM. Collagen tissue: implications of its response to stress in vitro. *Arch Phys Med Rehabil* 43: 461–466, 1962.

25. Sun JS, Tsuang YH, Liu TK, Hang YS, Cheng CK, and Lee WW. Viscoplasticity of rabbit skeletal muscle under dynamic cyclic loading. *Clin Biomech (Bristol, Avon)* 10: 258–262, 1995.

26. Warren CG, Lehmann JF, and Koblanski JN. Elongation of rat tail tendon: Effect of load and temperature. *Arch Phys Med Rehabil* 52: 465–474 passim, 1971.

27. Warren CG, Lehmann JF, and Koblanski JN. Heat and stretch procedures: an evaluation using rat tail tendon. *Arch Phys Med Rehabil* 57: 122–126, 1976.

28. Apostolopoulos N. Performance flexibility. In: *High-performance sports conditioning*. B Foran, ed. Champaign, IL: Human Kinetics 2001, pp 49–61.

29. Carpenter MG, Frank JS, and Silcher CP. Surface height effects on postural control: A hypothesis for a stiffness strategy for stance. *J Vestib Res* 9: 277–286, 1999.

30. Freitas SR, Mendes B, Le Sant G, Andrade RJ, Nordez A, and Milanovic Z. Can chronic stretching change the muscle-tendon mechanical properties? A review. *Scand J Med Sci Sports* 28(3): 794–806, 2017.

31. Trajano GS, Nosaka K, Seitz LB, and Blazevich AJ. Intermittent stretch reduces force and central drive more than continuous stretch. *Med Sci Sports Exerc* 46: 902–910, 2014.

32. Chtourou H, Aloui A, Hammouda O, Chaouachi A, Chamari K, and Souissi N. Effect of static and dynamic stretching on the diurnal variations of jump performance in soccer players. *PLoS One* 8: e70534, 2013.

33. McGill SM. *Low back disorders: evidence based prevention and rehabilitation.* Champaign, IL: Huma Kinetics Publishers, 2002.

34. Kraemer W, Fleck S, and Evans WJ. Strength and power training: physiological mechanisms of adaptation. *Sci Rev* 24: 363–397, 1990.

35. Kraemer WJ and Fleck S. Resistance training: Exercise prescription. *Phys SportsMed* 16: 69–81, 1988.

36. Kraemer WJ and Ratamess NA. Fundamentals of resistance training: Progression and exercise prescription. *Med Sci Sports Exerc* 36: 674–688, 2004.

37. Kubo K, Kanehisa H, and Fukunaga T. Effect of stretching training on the viscoelastic properties of human tendon structures in vivo. *J Appl Physiol* 92: 595–601, 2002.

38. Davis DS, Ashby PE, McHale KL, McQuain JA, and Wine JM. The effectiveness of 3 stretching techniques on hamstring flexibility using consistent stretching parameters. *J Strength Cond Res* 19: 27–32, 2005.

39. Yuktasir B and Kaya F. Investigation into the long term effects of static and PNF stretching exercises on range of motion and jump preformance. *J Bodyw Mov Ther* 13: 11–21, 2009.

40. Ben M and Harvey LA. Regular stretch does not increase muscle extensibility: A randomized controlled trial. *Scand J Med Sci Sports* 20 (1): 136–144, 2009.

41. Kubo K, Kanehisa H, and Fukunaga T. Effects of transient muscle contractions and stretching on the tendon structures in vivo. *Acta Physiol Scand* 175: 157–164, 2002.

42. Mahieu NN, McNair P, De MM, Stevens V, Blanckaert I, Smits N, and Witvrouw E. Effect of static and ballistic stretching on the muscle-tendon tissue properties. *Med Sci Sports Exerc* 39: 494–501, 2007.

43. Rancour J, Holmes CF, and Cipriani DJ. The effects of intermittent stretching following a 4-week static stretching protocol: A randomized trial. *J Strength Cond Res* 23: 2217–2222, 2009.

44. Ross MD. Effect of a 15-day pragmatic hamstring stretching program on hamstring flexibility and single hop for distance test performance. *Res Sports Med* 15: 271–281, 2007.

45. Ylinen J, Kankainen T, Kautiainen H, Rezasoltani A, Kuukkanen T, and Hakkinen A. Effect of stretching on hamstring muscle compliance. *J Rehabil Med* 41: 80–84, 2009.

46. Wallin D, Ekblom B, Grahn R, and Nordenborg T. Improvement of muscle flexibility. A comparison between two techniques. *Am J Sports Med* 13: 263–268, 1985.

47. Inami T, Shimizu T, Baba R, and Nakagaki A. Acute changes in autonomic nerve activity during passive static stretching. *Am J Sports Sci Med* 2: 166–170, 2014.

48. Farinatti PT, Brandao C, Soares PP, and Duarte AF. Acute effects of stretching exercise on the heart rate variability in subjects with low flexibility levels. *J Strength Cond Res* 25: 1579–1585, 2011.

49. Volek J, Kraemer W, Bush J, Incledon T, and Boetes M. Testosterone and cortisol in relationship to dietary nutrients and resistance exercise. *J Appl Physiol* 82: 49–54, 1997.

50. Gonzalez AM, Hoffman JR, Townsend JR, Jajtner AR, Boone CH, Beyer KS, Baker KM, Wells AJ, Mangine GT, Robinson EHt, Church DD, Oliveira LP, Willoughby DS, Fukuda DH, and Stout JR. Intramuscular anabolic signaling and endocrine response following high volume and high intensity resistance exercise protocols in trained men. *Physiol Rep* 3: 127–133, 2015.

51. Balaji PA, Varne SR, and Ali SS. Physiological effects of yogic practices and transcendental meditation in health and disease. *N Am J Med Sci* 4: 442–448, 2012.

52. Coulter D. *Anatomy of hatha yoga*. Honesdale, PA: Body and Breath, 2001.

53. Dane S, Caliskan E, Karasen M, and Oztasan N. Effects of unilateral nostril breathing on blood pressure and heart rate in right-handed healthy subjects. *Int J Neurosci* 112: 97–102, 2002.

54. Campbell EJM. Accessory muscles. In: *The respiratory muscles mechanics and neural control*. Philadelphia, PA: WB Saunders 1970, pp 181–193.

55. Roaf R. *Posture*. New York: Academic Press, 1977.

56. Hamilton AR, Beck KL, Kaulbach J, Kenny M, Basset FA, Di Santo MC, and Behm DG. Breathing techniques affect female but not male hip flexion range of motion. *J Strength Cond Res* 29: 3197–3205, 2015.

57. Borsa PA, Sauers EL, and Herling DE. Patterns of glenohumeral joint laxity and stiffness in healthy men and women. *Med Sci Sports Exerc* 32: 1685–1690, 2000.

58. McHugh MP, Kremenic IJ, Fox MB, and Gleim GW. The role of mechanical and neural restraints to joint range of motion during passive stretch. *Med Sci Sports Exerc* 30: 928–932, 1998.

59. Seals DR, Suwarno NO, and Dempsey JA. Influence of lung volume on sympathetic nerve discharge in normal humans. *Circ Res* 67: 130–141, 1990.

60. Fasen JM, O'Connor AM, Schwartz SL, Watson JO, Plastaras CT, Garvan CW, Bulcao C, Johnson SC, and Akuthota V. A randomized controlled trial of hamstring stretching: comparison of four techniques. *J Strength Cond Res* 23: 660–667, 2009.

61. Huang SY, Di Santo M, Wadden KP, Cappa DF, Alkanani T, and Behm DG. Short-duration massage at the hamstrings musculotendinous junction induces greater range of motion. *J Strength Cond Res* 24: 1917–1924, 2010.

62. Noonan TJ, Best TM, Seaber AV, and Garrett WE, Jr. Thermal effects on skeletal muscle tensile behavior. *Am J Sports Med* 21: 517–522, 1993.

63. Rigby BJ. The effect of mechanical extension upon the thermal stability of collagen. *Biochim Biophys Acta* 79: 634–636, 1964.

64. Lehmann JF and DeLateur BJ. Diathermy and superficial heat, laser, and cold therapy. In: *Krusen's handbook of physical medicine and rehabilitation*. Philadelphia: Saunders, 1990, pp 285–367.

65. Mason T and Rigby BJ. Thermal transition in collagen. *Biochim Biophys Acta* 66: 448–450, 1963.

66. Rigby BJ, Hirai N, Spikes JD, and Eyring H. The mechanical properties of rat tail tendon. *J Gen Physiol* 43: 265–283, 1959.

67. Sechrist WC and Stull GA. Effect of mild activity, heat applications, and cold applications on range of joint movement. *Am Correct Ther J* 23: 120–123, 1969.

68. Lentell G, Hetherington T, Eagan J, and Morgan M. The use of thermal agents to influence the effectiveness of a low-load prolonged stretch. *J Orthop Sports Phys Ther* 16: 200–207, 1992.

69. Wessling KC, DeVane DA, and Hylton CR. Effects of static stretch versus static stretch and ultrasound combined on triceps surae muscle extensibility in healthy women. *Phys Ther* 67: 674–679, 1987.

70. Peres SE, Draper DO, Knight KL, and Richard MD. Pulsed shortwave diathermy and prolonged stretch increase dorsiflexion range of motion more than prolonged stretch alone. *J Athl Train* 2: S49, 2001.

71. Sawyer PC, Uhl TL, Mattacola CG, Johnson DL, and Yates JW. Effects of moist heat on hamstring flexibility and muscle temperature. *J Strength Cond Res* 17: 285–290, 2003.

72. Henricson AS, Fredriksson K, Persson I, Pereira R, Rostedt Y, and Westlin NE. The effect of heat and stretching on the range of hip motion*. *J Orthop Sports Phys Ther* 6: 110–115, 1984.

73. Hardy M and Woodall W. Therapeutic effects of heat, cold, and stretch on connective tissue. *J Hand Ther* 11: 148–156, 1998.

74. Lehmann JF, Masock AJ, Warren CG, and Koblanski JN. Effect of therapeutic temperatures on tendon extensibility. *Arch Phys Med Rehabil* 51: 481–487, 1970.

75. Sapega AA, Quedenfeld TC, Moyer RA, and Butler RA. Biophysical factors in range-of-motion exercise. *Phys Sportsmed* 9: 57–65, 1981.

76. Newton RA. Effects of vapocoolants on passive hip flexion in healthy subjects. *Phys Ther* 65: 1034–1036, 1985.

77. Cornelius Wl and Jackson A. The effescts of cryotherapy and PNF on hip extensor flexibility. *Athl Train* 19: 183–199, 1984.

78. Cornelius WL. Exercise beneficials to the hip but questionable for the knee. *NSCA J* 5: 40–41, 1984.

79. Minton J. 1992 student writing contest-1st runner-up: A comparison of thermotherapy and cryotherapy in enhancing supine, extended-leg, hip flexion. *J Athl Train* 28: 172–176, 1993.

80. Rosenberg BS, Cornelius WL, and Jackson AW. The effects of cryotherapy and PNF stretching techniques on hip extensor flexibility in elderly females. *J Phys Educ Sport Sci* 2: 31–36, 1990.

81. Burke DG, Holt LE, Rasmussen R, MacKinnon NC, Vossen JF, and Pelham TW. Effects of hot or cold water immersion and modified proprioceptive neuromuscular facilitation flexibility exercise on hamstring length. *J Athl Train* 36: 16–19, 2001.

82. Behm DG and Sale DG. Velocity specificity of resistance training. *Sports Med* 15: 374–388, 1993.

83. Kibele A, Granacher U, Muehlbauer T, and Behm DG. Stable, unstable and metastable states of equilibrium: definitions and applications to human movement. *J Sports Sci Med* 14: 885–887, 2015.

7

STRETCHING EFFECTS ON INJURY REDUCTION AND HEALTH

The triumvirate of reasons for stretching over the decades has been to increase range of motion (ROM), improve performance, and decrease the chances for injury. The research is overwhelming that we can increase flexibility with stretching. However, the next two traditional reasons for stretching are less clear. We discuss in Chapter 8 how an acute session of prolonged static stretching might actually impair performance rather than improve it. The contention that stretching reduces injuries is also mired in controversy.

An Australian researcher, Rodney Pope, is well cited for his work in the area. Pope et al. (1) investigated 1093 Australian army recruits during 12 weeks of military training and found a significant correlation between dorsiflexion ROM and injury incidence. The injuries they followed were ankle sprains, tibia or foot stress fractures, tibial periostitis, Achilles tendonitis, and anterior tibial component syndrome. Poor flexibility was associated with 2.5 times the risk for such injuries compared with average dorsiflexion ROM and 8 times the risk compared with people with a high level of flexibility. However, the stretch-training programme had no significant effect on the incidence of these injuries. Do these two statements not conflict with each other? Not entirely! The amount of flexibility is an intrinsic factor (something that you have), whereas stretching is an extrinsic factor (something that you do). So, in the first Pope study, in general if you had better dorsiflexion ROM then you were less likely to get injured. However, doing a stretching programme did not change the risks to a significant degree. In a similar later study, Pope et al. (2) involved 1538 Australian army recruits who performed one stretch each for six lower leg muscles every second day. The stretch-training programme did not produce a clinically worthwhile reduction in lower limb injury risk. Injuries included lower body stress fractures, muscle strains, ligament sprains, periostitis, tendonitis, meniscal lesions, compartment syndromes, and bursitis, among others. Thus, neither of Pope's studies showed an extrinsic effect of stretching on injury incidence. Small and colleagues (3) reported similar results in their review. Four randomized clinical trials found that static stretching was ineffective in reducing the incidence of exercise-related injury, and one of three controlled clinical trials indicated that static stretching decreased the incidence of exercise-related injury. However, three of the seven studies reported reductions in musculotendinous and ligament injuries, although there were no statistically significant reductions in the all-injury risk. Small et al. concluded that there was moderate-to-strong evidence that static stretching does not reduce overall injury rates, but may reduce musculotendinous injuries. Weldon and Hill (4) said they could not make a definitive statement due to the paucity of well-controlled studies at that time. They went as far to say that the scant evidence before 2003 would suggest that pre-exercise stretching may actually increase the risk of injury. However, they did not seem that convinced because they also offered that scientific and clinical evidence indicated that stretching in the post-exercise period (cool-down) should increase the energy-absorbing capabilities of the musculotendinous unit (MTU), reducing the risk of injury. Shrier (5), in his review, also indicated that stretching before an event will not reduce injuries. Just to confuse the public a bit more, a review by Woods et al. (6) contradicted the earlier reviews by stating that using particular techniques or protocols would provide a reduction in injuries. They indicated that by elongating muscle length to provide a greater ROM this would lead to fewer MTU injuries. They recommended that it was important to ensure an anterior pelvic tilt with the hip at 90° of flexion when stretching the hamstrings.

The confusion resides in whether the reviews are examining all-injury risk versus MTU injury risk. How can pre-event stretching be expected to reduce lower body fractures, meniscal lesions, bursitis, or other afflictions? Will stretching reduce overtraining effects typical of long-distance runners and cyclists? It is unlikely, according to the literature. But, if stretching can improve the energy-absorbing capabilities of the MTU, then you might expect a positive trend for stretching to prevent musculotendinous injuries, especially those caused by high loads associated with rapid force absorption such as sprinting and agility.

In the latest review by Behm et al. (7), Dr Malachy McHugh (a proud Irishman working in New York) was responsible for the section on injury incidence. In his review of stretching articles investigating injury evidence, he found that eight studies showed some effectiveness of stretching, whereas four showed no effect. There was no evidence that stretching negatively influences (increases) injury risk. Only two of five studies that stretched for less than 5 minutes indicated reduced injury risk whereas five of six stretching studies with more than 5 minutes showed an injury incidence benefit for stretching. Only two of five stretching studies showed injury reduction benefits for endurance sports or military training, which typically involves overuse injuries. Five of six studies showed fewer injuries with sprint running type of sports. The effectiveness of stretching for sprint activities could be related to the high tensile demands placed on the MTU with the stretch-shortening cycle. Witvrouw et al. (8) suggest that, by increasing the compliance of the tendon, the tissue will have greater energy-absorbing capacity. However, as static stretching may not be as effective as ballistic stretching for decreasing tendon stiffness, they recommend including ballistic stretching within the warm-up. Fradkin et al. (9), in another review, reported that three of the five studies they reviewed showed significant injury prevention benefits with little evidence to suggest stretching was harmful in terms of inflicting injuries. Furthermore, most research (except for one study (10)) reports that stretching does not reduce muscle soreness or other symptoms of muscle damage. Stretching also does not improve recovery from fatigue and may actually inhibit recovery (11). Although it is a very common practice, one article reports that acute static and PNF stretching did not prevent the frequency of muscle cramping (12). Thus, in summary, pre-activity stretching of ≥5 min should be more beneficial for injury prevention with sprint running, but less effective with endurance-type running activities (13) (including military training) which tend to lead to overuse injuries. As workplace injuries are also often overuse injuries, the recommendation to stretch at work may not be as effective as is often promoted. Behm et al. (7) report the studies in their review indicate a 54% risk reduction in acute muscle and tendon injuries associated with stretching.

However, Chapter 8 will emphasize to the reader that more than 60 seconds of static stretching per muscle group without a full warm-up could lead to performance impairments. It is important to note that the research says "per muscle group". To reduce the risk of injury incidence you should stretch more than one muscle group. So, to reduce lower body injuries you might want to static stretch the hip flexors and extensors, knee extensors and flexors, abductors and adductors, dorsiflexors, plantar flexors, and ankle evertors for 60 seconds for "each", resulting in perhaps 9 minutes of lower body stretching.

Physiological rationale for stretch-induced injury reduction

Why would stretching have an effect on injury incidence, especially with higher speed running activities such as sprinting or change of direction (i.e. agility)? Unfortunately, most of the studies that investigate injury risk have not provided a rationale for reduced injuries (14). Theoretically, it is possible that stretching makes the MTU more compliant (15,16), increased compliance shifts the angle–torque relationship to allow greater relative force production at longer muscle lengths (15,17), and thus the improved resistance to excessive muscle elongation may decrease the susceptibility to muscle strain. Similarly, stretching for 5 minutes can increase tendon compliance and decrease hysteresis (18), which would also allow the tendon to absorb forces over a more extended duration, decreasing the stress on this connective tissue and minimizing the possibility of a strain. On the other hand, a competing rationale could be that increased muscle force output from a lengthened muscle could increase the likelihood of injury. However, this rationale would not apply to the risk of other injuries such as ligament sprains, skeletal fractures or overuse injuries. In general, the ability of the MTU to better absorb force perturbations, whether due to less MTU stiffness (greater compliance) or higher force capabilities at longer muscle lengths, should reduce injuries, especially with high forces and torques associated with sprinting and agility. Dr McHugh provided the following theory and application in a personal correspondence:

> Muscle strains can occur during concentric contractions and can occur at short muscle lengths. For example, in the days when soccer balls were made with leather and the ball became much heavier in wet conditions it was common to see rectus femoris strains in players kicking a ball (often complete ruptures). At the point of impact with the ball the rectus femoris MTU is shortening (knee is extending, hip is flexing). However, the brain has programmed the body to expect impact with an object with a particular mass. The actual mass is in fact greater than expected due to the wet conditions. At the point of impact with the ball, the contractile and non-contractile elements are shortening synchronously to optimize the impulse imparted on the ball. When the resistance to movement provided by the ball is greater than expected this subtly changes the internal muscle tendon mechanics; at the knee quadriceps and patellar tendon recoil act to extend the knee, if the rate of knee extension is slowed by a heavier than expected ball this will change the loading at the muscle tendon junction (in simplistic terms the tendon is now pulling on the muscle fibers mores than the bone because an external force has slowed joint movement). I think that anything that disrupts the interaction between tendon and muscle mechanics during forceful stretch-shortening cycle movements can cause injury to the muscle-tendon unit.

Dr McHugh continued as follows:

> I think the ability of a contracted muscle to absorb sudden tensile loads is important in the mechanism of muscle strains. If an isometrically contracted muscle is stretched suddenly (even a little stretch) there is a large increase in force that is due to the mechanical resistance of the MTU (19,20). In many cases, due to the very brief onset, the stretch reflex or other neural changes cannot contribute. I think if the contractile component is able to resist the elongation and impart it to the tendon the muscle will be protected from potential strain injury. Stretching might impact this (albeit in a small way) by allowing greater myofilament overlap at longer muscle lengths than was achievable before the acute bout of stretching, thus allowing the muscle tendon unit elongation to be transferred to the non-contractile component.

Stretching effects on posture, low back pain, and compensatory overuse syndromes

A lack of flexibility in the pelvis, back, or other joints can lead to poor posture (21). We strive to keep our centre of gravity over our base of support (equilibrium or balance) or we want to be able to temporarily move our centre of gravity outside our base of support and return to a balanced position (metastability) (22) when reaching or moving. Poor flexibility leading to poor posture, as seen with rounded shoulders, or insufficient lumbar spinal curves can hamper our balance or movement capabilities. We then try to overcompensate by engaging other muscles and joints to achieve these functions. The shortened or inflexible muscles may also atrophy and become weaker, leading to muscle imbalances (agonist to antagonist muscle activity or prime mover to synergist muscle activity). As the other muscles or joints may not be efficient at achieving these movements, they may be susceptible to fatigue, overuse, and perhaps eventual injury. A combination of flexibility training, muscle strengthening, and movement re-education might be needed to return the body to proper functioning and reduce the possibility of pain, discomfort, and possible injury with these movements.

The role of improving back flexibility to reduce the incidence of low back pain is controversial. It seems that both ends of the spectrum – lack of back flexibility or mobility (23–25) and excessive spinal mobility (26) – can contribute to back problems. However, others have reported that tight hip flexors (27), lack of lumbar or hip motion (27), or thoracic mobility (28) was not related to low back pain. None the less, many authors emphasize the need for adequate back or trunk mobility in order to ensure proper mechanical functioning (29), otherwise the excessive bending movements on individual vertebrae can lead to an increased injury risk (30). It is suggested, by many researchers and organizations, that adequate flexibility can reduce the incidence and severity of low back pain (31–36). Based on the evidence for and against the protection of lower back problems with greater back ROM (37–39), Stu McGill suggests that trunk stretching should not emphasize maximum ROM, and torso flexibility exercises should be limited to unloaded flexion and extension, ensure adequate hip and knee flexibility, so that the back does not have to overcompensate (compensatory relative flexibility (40)) for other inflexible joints, and finally the first concern should be to improve the strength and endurance of the back before incorporating back or trunk flexibility programmes.

Effects of immobilization on flexibility

When an individual is injured and subjected to immobilization, the consequences can include muscle atrophy (41–43), decreases in dynamic (42) and static strength (44,45), muscle activation (46,47), reflex potentiation (48), and maximum motor unit firing rates (49,50), as well as increases in the duration of twitch contractile properties (44,45,50). In addition, immobilization can adversely affect flexibility (51). Prolonged immobilization with the muscle in a shortened position can decrease the number of sarcomeres in series, shortening muscle fibre length (52–54). Fortunately, this sarcomere loss can be rapidly regenerated once normal activity and muscle lengthening occur (52–54). Conversely, if a muscle is immobilized in a lengthened position, additional sarcomeres are added (53). Unfortunately, the biomechanics of our joints and muscles dictate that, when one muscle is in a lengthened position, the other is typically in a shortened position, so there is no strategy that can benefit both muscles at the same time.

Another factor contributing to a more inflexible muscle with immobilization would be a relative increase in connective tissue, because connective tissue degrades at a slower rate than muscle tissue, contributing to a stiffer muscle (53,54). In addition, there is reported to be a more acute angle of collagen to the axis of the muscle fibres compared with healthy muscle (55) which would also affect stiffness. Third, immobilization reduces the water and glycosaminoglycan content of connective tissue, decreasing the distance between collagen fibres and resulting in abnormal cross-linkages that limit extensibility of the tissue (56,57). Stretching tends to counter these deleterious effects (58). However, an immobilized limb in a cast may be difficult to stretch in order to prevent or reduce the decreased extensibility. A counter-measure that may be incorporated while the muscle is still immobilized is to stretch the contralateral muscle or actually any other muscle. Unilateral stretching of the hamstrings has improved the ROM of the contralateral hip flexors (59). Furthermore, stretching either the shoulders or the adductor (groin) muscles resulted in improved ROM in the hip flexors and shoulders, respectively (60). So, stretch your upper body and your lower body becomes more flexible or stretch your lower body and your upper body becomes more flexible. This is important information for individuals who are immobilized. Just like cross-education (strength increase in contralateral muscle after unilateral training) (61–64) is important to preserve strength in an immobilized muscle, stretching unaffected muscles should help to preserve flexibility or at least help to minimize loss of flexibility during immobilization.

Stretching effects on dysmenorrhoea

Another painful or uncomfortable condition that may be alleviated by stretching is dysmenorrhoea (65). Dysmenorrhoea is greater than the normal pain or discomfort associated with menstruation. Although it can be attributed in some cases to abnormal oestrogen–progesterone balance, poor posture due to shortening of uterine connective tissue, which affects the pelvic posterior tilt, has also been postulated (35,66). Static stretching of the pelvis on a consistent basis has been reported to alleviate or reduce dysmenorrhoea (66–68). It is speculated that the stretching decreases the stiffness or restrictions of the fascia and ligaments, relieving the compression and irritation of the affected nerves (69,70).

Stretching effects on the cardiovascular system

Stretching can have both positive and negative effects on the cardiovascular system. Static stretching for 1–4 minutes enhanced blood flow to the stretched muscle for 10 minutes after stretching (71). However, static stretching also increases heart rate, blood pressure, and rate pressure product (rate pressure product [RPP] = heart rate [HR] × systolic blood pressure [BP]: a measure of myocardial workload), especially when Valsalva's manoeuvre (exhaling against a closed glottis) was used during the stretching procedure. This increased cardiovascular strain could be dangerous for people with heart and cardiovascular problems (72). Furthermore, it has been shown that poor flexibility is associated with greater age-related arterial stiffening (73). Remember that associations and correlations are not causative. This means that improving your flexibility will not necessarily decrease arterial stiffness. It may just mean that people with stiff arteries have not been active throughout their lives and poor flexibility is just one sign that their sedentary lifestyle has contributed to possible arteriosclerosis. However, cyclical stretching can have positive effects on the cell shape, cytoplasmic organization, and intracellular processes of vascular smooth muscle cells. When stretching, you are unlikely to stretch the arteries directly but, as the vasculature cytoskeleton and contractile proteins are associated with and embedded into the extracellular matrix (ECM), stretching can move, deform, or place stress on the surrounding ECM, and thus stimulate the vascular cell membrane receptors (74). So, while we normally think of aerobic exercise and nutrition as being the most important factors for cardiovascular health, stretching can also contribute to a healthy cardiovascular system.

Summary

Generally, there is no strong evidence for stretching programmes to reduce the incidence of all-cause injuries. However, there is more convincing evidence that a stretch-training programme can reduce the incidence of musculotendinous and ligamentous injuries, especially with more powerful actions such as sprinting and changing direction (agility). Flexibility training may increase the energy-absorbing capability of the MTU because a more compliant tissue will absorb these forces over a more prolonged duration. It is unlikely that neural reflexes contribute greatly to this improved protection because the unexpected loads or torques from a slip, fall, or collision may be too rapid to be affected by a reflex response. Chronic problems such as low back pain might be positively affected by stretch training because the increased flexibility may improve hip/pelvic orientation, affecting spinal curves and alleviating back pain and compensatory overuse syndromes. Similarly, stretching may decrease the discomfort of dysmenorrhoea by reducing fascia and ligament stiffness and restrictions. It is important to stretch an immobilized limb because there can be a shortening of the muscle primarily due to abnormal cross-linkages and, in very prolonged cases, to decreases in sarcomeres in series. Even stretching another muscle such as the contralateral homologous or heterologous muscle can help maintain a certain degree of ROM in the affected muscle. Although enhanced flexibility correlates with decreased arterial stiffness and stretching can increase blood flow to the stretched muscle, individuals with cardiovascular diseases must be cautious due to stretch-induced increases in the rate pressure product (heart rate × blood pressure: a measure of cardiac workload or demand).

References

1. Pope R, Herbert R, and Kirwan J. Effects of ankle dorsiflexion range and pre-exercise calf muscle stretching on injury risk in army recruits. *Aust J Physiother* 44: 165–177, 1998.
2. Pope R, Herbert R, Kirwan J, and Graham B. A randomized trial of preexercise stretching for prevention of lower-limb injury. *Med Sci Sport Exer* 32: 271, 2000.
3. Small K, Mc Naughton L, and Matthews M. A systematic review into the efficacy of static stretching as part of a warm-up for the prevention of exercise-related injury. *Res Sports Med* 16: 213–231, 2008.
4. Weldon SM and Hill RH. The efficacy of stretching for prevention of exercise-related injury: A systematic review of the literature. *Man Ther* 8: 141–150, 2003.
5. Shrier I. Does stretching improve performance? A systematic and critical review of the literature 39. *Clin J Sport Med* 14: 267–273, 2004.
6. Woods K, Bishop P, and Jones E. Warm-up and stretching in the prevention of muscular injury. *Sports Med* 37: 1089–1099, 2007.
7. Behm DG, Blazevich AJ, Kay AD, and McHugh M. Acute effects of muscle stretching on physical performance, range of motion, and injury incidence in healthy active individuals: A systematic review. *Appl Physiol Nutr Metab* 41: 1–11, 2016.
8. Witvrouw E, Mahieu N, Roosen P, and McNair P. The role of stretching in tendon injuries. *Br J Sports Med* 41: 224–226, 2007.
9. Fradkin AJ, Gabbe BJ, and Cameron PA. Does warming up prevent injury in sport? The evidence from randomised controlled trials? *J Sci Med Sport* 9: 214–220, 2006.
10. Chen HM, Wang HH, Chen CH, and Hu HM. Effectiveness of a stretching exercise program on low back pain and exercise self-efficacy among nurses in Taiwan: A randomized clinical trial. *Pain Manag Nurs* 15: 283–291, 2014.
11. Eguchi Y, Jinde M, Murooka K, Konno Y, Ohta M, and Yamato H. Stretching versus transitory icing: Which is the more effective treatment for attenuating muscle fatigue after repeated manual labor? *Eur J Appl Physiol* 114: 2617–2623, 2014.
12. Miller KC, Harsen JD, and Long BC. Prophylactic stretching does not reduce cramp susceptibility. *Muscle Nerve* 57 (3): 473–477, 2017.
13. Baxter C, Mc Naughton LR, Sparks A, Norton L, and Bentley D. Impact of stretching on the performance and injury risk of long-distance runners. *Res Sports Med* 25: 78–90, 2017.
14. McHugh MP and Cosgrave CH. To stretch or not to stretch: The role of stretching in injury prevention and performance. *Scand J Med Sci Sports* 20: 169–181, 2010.
15. McHugh MP and Nesse M. Effect of stretching on strength loss and pain after eccentric exercise. *Med Sci Sports Exerc* 40: 566–573, 2008.
16. Toft E, Espersen GT, Külund S, Sinkjër T, and Hornemann BC. Passive tension of the ankle before and after stretching. *Am J Sport Med* 17: 489–494, 1989.

17. Herda TJ, Cramer JT, Ryan ED, McHugh MP, and Stout JR. Acute effects of static versus dynamic stretching on isometric peak torque, electromyography, and mechanomyography of the biceps femoris muscle. *J Strength Cond Res* 22: 809–817, 2008.

18. Kubo K, Kanehisa H, and Fukunaga T. Effects of transient muscle contractions and stretching on the tendon structures in vivo. *Acta Physiol Scand* 175: 157–164, 2002.

19. McHugh M and Hogan D. Effect of knee flexion angle on active joint stiffness. *Acta Physiol Scand* 180: 249–254, 2004.

20. Webber S and Kriellaars D. Neuromuscular factors contributing to in vivo eccentric moment generation. *J Appl Physiol (1985)* 83: 40–45, 1997.

21. Corbin CB and Noble L. Flexibility: A major component of physical fitness. *JPN Phys Educ Recreation* 6: 23–24, 57–60, 1980.

22. Kibele A, Granacher U, Muehlbauer T, and Behm DG. Stable, unstable and metastable states of equilibrium: Definitions and applications to human movement. *J Sports Sci Med* 14: 885–887, 2015.

23. Burton AK, Tillotson KM, and Troup, JD. Variation in lumbar sagittal mobility with low-back trouble. *Spine* 6: 584–590, 1989.

24. Curtis L, Mayer TG, and Gatchel RJ. Physical progress and residual impairment quantification after functional restoration. Part III: Isokinetic and isoinertial lifting capacity. *Spine (Phila Pa 1976)* 19: 401–405, 1994.

25. Waddell G, Somerville D, Henderson I, and Newton M. Objective clinical evaluation of physical impairment in chronic low back pain. *Spine (Phila Pa 1976)* 17: 617–628, 1992.

26. Howes RG and Isdale IC. The non-myotendinous force transmission. *Rheumatol Phys Med* 11: 72–77, 1971.

27. Esola MA, McClure PW, Fitzgerald GK, and Siegler S. Analysis of lumbar spine and hip motion during forward bending in subjects with and without a history of low back pain. *Spine (Phila Pa 1976)* 21: 71–78, 1996.

28. Lundberg G and Gerdle B. Correlations between joint and spinal mobility, spinal sagittal configuration, segmental mobility, segmental pain, symptoms and disabilities in female homecare personnel. *Scand J Rehabil Med* 32: 124–133, 2000.

29. Farfan HF. The biomechanical advantage of lordosis and hip extension for upright activity. Man as compared with other anthropoids. *Spine (Phila Pa 1976)* 3: 336–342, 1978.

30. Dolan P and Adams MA. Influence of lumbar and hip mobility on the bending stresses acting on the lumbar spine. *Clin Biomech* 8: 185–192, 1993.

31. American College of Sports Medicine. ACSM's guidelines for exercise testing and prescription. *Med Sci Sport Exer* 6: 158–164, 2000.

32. Cailliet R. *Low back pain syndrome*. Philadelphia, PA: FA Davis, 1988.

33. Deyo RA, Walsh NE, Martin DC, Schoenfeld LS, and Ramamurthy S. A controlled trial of transcutaneous electrical nerve stimulation (TENS) and exercise for chronic low back pain. *N Engl J Med* 322: 1627–1634, 1990.

34. Locke JC. Stretching away from back pain, injury. *Occup Health Saf* 52: 8–13, 1983.

35. Rasch PJ. *Kinesiology and applied anatomy*. Philadelphia, PA: Lea & Febiger, 1989.

36. Russell GS and Highland, TR. *Care of the lower back*. Columbia, MO: Spine, 1990.

37. Battie MC, Bigos SJ, Fisher LD, Spengler DM, Hansson TH, Nachemson AL, and Wortley MD. The role of spinal flexibility in back pain complaints within industry: A prospective study. *Spine* 8: 768–773, 1990.

38. Battie MC, Bigos SJ, Sheehy A, and Wortley MD. Spinal flexibility and individual factors that influence it. *Phys Ther* 67: 653–658, 1987.

39. McGill SM. Stability: From biomechanical concepts to chiropractic practice. *J Can Chirop Assn* 2: 75–88, 1999.

40. Sahrmann SA. *Diagnosis and treatment of movement impairment syndromes.* St Louis, MO: Mosby Publishers 2002.
41. Dudley GA, Duvoisin MR, Adams GR, Meyer RA, Belew AH, and Buchanan P. Adaptations to unilateral lower limb suspensions in humans. *Aviat Space Envir Md* 63: 678–683, 1992.
42. Halkjaer-Kristensen J and Ingemann-Hansen T. Wasting of the human quadriceps muscle after knee ligament injuries. IV dynamic and static muscle function. *Scand J Rehab Med Suppl* 13: 29–37, 1985.
43. Halkjaer-Kristensen J and Ingemann-Hansen T. Wasting of the human quadriceps muscle after ligament injuries. I anthropometrical consequences. *Scand J Rehab Med Suppl* 13: 5–10, 1985.
44. White MJ and Davies CTM. The effects of immobilization, after lower leg fracture, on the contractile properties of human triceps surae. *Clin Sci* 66: 277–282, 1984.
45. White MJ, Davies CTM, and Brooksby P. The effects of short-term voluntary immobilization on the contractile properties of the human triceps surae. *J Gen Physiol* 69: 21–27, 1984.
46. Duchateau J and Hainaut K. Effects of immobilization on electromyogram power spectrum changes during fatigue. *Eur J Appl Physiol O* 63: 458–462, 1991.
47. Fuglsang-Fredriksen A and Scheel U. Transient decrease in number of motor units after immobilisation in man. *J Neurol Neurosur Psychiatry* 41: 924–929, 1978.
48. Sale DG, McComas AJ, MacDougall JD, and Upton ARM. Neuromuscular adaptation in human thenar muscles following strength training and immobilization. *J Appl Physiol* 53: 419–424, 1982.
49. Duchateau J and Hainaut K. Electrical and mechanical changes in immobilized human muscle. *J Appl Physiol* 62: 2168–2173, 1987.
50. Duchateau J and Hainaut K. Effects of immobilization on contractile properties recruitment and firing rates of human motor units. *J Physiol* 422: 55–65, 1990.
51. Behm DG. Debilitation to adaptation. *J Strength Cond Res* 7: 65–75, 1993.
52. Goldspink G, Tabary C, Tabary JC, Tardieu C, and Tardieu G. Effect of denervation on the adaptation of sarcomere number and muscle extensibility to the functional length of the muscle. *J Physiol* 236: 733–742, 1974.
53. Tabary JC, Tabary C, Tardieu C, Tardieu G, and Goldspink G. Physiological and structural changes in the cat's soleus muscle due to immobilization at different lengths by plaster casts. *J Physiol* 224: 231–244, 1972.
54. Tabary JC, Tardieu C, Tabary C, Lombard M, Gagnard L, and Tardieu G. [Readaptation of the number of sarcomeres in series in isolated soleus fibers after neurectomy]. *J Physiol (Paris)* 65(Suppl 3): 509A, 1972.
55. Goldspink G and Williams PE. The nature of the increased passive resistance in muscle immobilization of the mouse soleus muscle [proceedings]. *J Physiol* 289: 55P, 1979.
56. Akeson WH, Amiel D, and Woo S. Immobility effects on synovial joints the pathomechanics of joint contraction. *Biorheology* 1/2: 95–110, 1980.
57. McDonough AL. Effects of immobilization and exercise on articular cartilage: A review of the literature. *J Orthop Sport Phys Therapy* 1: 2–5, 1981.
58. Ahtikoski AM, Koskinen SO, Virtanen P, Kovanen V, and Takala TE. Regulation of synthesis of fibrillar collagens in rat skeletal muscle during immobilization in shortened and lengthened positions. *Acta Physiol Scand* 172: 131–140, 2001.
59. Chaouachi A, Padulo J, Kasmi S, Othmen AB, Chatra M, and Behm DG. Unilateral static and dynamic hamstrings stretching increases contralateral hip flexion range of motion. *Clin Physiol Funct Imaging* 37: 23–29, 2017.

60. Behm DG, Cavanaugh T, Quigley P, Reid JC, Nardi PS, and Marchetti PH. Acute bouts of upper and lower body static and dynamic stretching increase non-local joint range of motion. *Eur J Appl Physiol* 116: 241–249, 2016.

61. Hellebrandt FA. Cross education: Ipsilateral and contralateral effects of unimanual training. *J Appl Physiol* 4: 136–144, 1951.

62. Hortobagyi T. Cross education and the human central nervous system: Mechanisms of unilateral interventions producing contralateral adaptations. *IEEE Eng Med Biol* 24: 22–28, 2005.

63. Shima N, Ishida K, Katayama K, Morotome Y, Sato Y, and Miyamura M. Cross education of muscular strength during unilateral resistance training and detraining. *Eur J Appl Physiol* 86: 287–294, 2002.

64. Zhou S. Chronic neural adaptations to unilateral exercise: Mechanisms of cross education. *Exerc Sport Sci Rev* 28: 177–184, 2000.

65. Alter MJ. *Science of flexibility*. Champaign, IL: Human Kinetics, 1996.

66. Golub LJ. Exercises that alleviate primary dysmenorrhea. *Contemp Ob Gyn* 5: 51–59, 1987.

67. Golub LJ, Menduke H, and Lang WR. Exercise and dysmenorrhea in young teenagers: A 3-year study. *Obstet Gynecol* 32: 508–511, 1968.

68. Golub LJ, Lang WR, and Menduke, H. Dysmenorrhea in high school and college girls: Relationship to sports participation. *Western J Surg Obstet Gynecol* 3: 163–165, 1958.

69. Billing HE. Dysmenorrhea: The result of a postural defect. *Arch Surg* 5: 611–613, 1943.

70. Billing HE. Fascial stretching. *J Phys Ment Rehabil* 1: 4–8, 1951.

71. Kruse NT and Scheuermann BW. Effect of self-administered stretching on NIRS-measured oxygenation dynamics. *Clin Physiol Funct Imaging* 36: 126–133, 2016.

72. Lima TP, Farinatti PT, Rubini EC, Silva EB, and Monteiro WD. Hemodynamic responses during and after multiple sets of stretching exercises performed with and without the Valsalva maneuver. *Clinics (Sao Paulo)* 70: 333–338, 2015.

73. Yamamoto K, Kawano H, Gando Y, Iemitsu M, Murakami H, Sanada K, Tanimoto M, Ohmori Y, Higuchi M, Tabata I, and Miyachi M. Poor trunk flexibility is associated with arterial stiffening. *Am J Physiol Heart Circ Physiol* 297: H1314–H1318, 2009.

74. Halka AT, Turner NJ, Carter A, Ghosh J, Murphy MO, Kirton JP, Kielty CM, and Walker MG. The effects of stretch on vascular smooth muscle cell phenotype in vitro. *Cardiovasc Pathol* 17: 98–102, 2008.

8

DOES STRETCHING AFFECT PERFORMANCE?

Static and proprioceptive neuromuscular facilitation stretching

At least from the mid-twentieth century, stretching was believed to enhance performance. An early study by the renowned George Dintiman reported that stretch training enhanced sprint speed (1). However, various studies have indicated no beneficial effects of stretch training on the oxygen cost of running (3 days/week for 10 weeks) (2), drop jumps (4 days/week for 6 weeks) (3), vertical jumps (4 days/week for 6 weeks) (4), or sprint speed (4), whereas static stretching 2 days/week for 8 weeks did improve rebound bench-press performance (5). Lately the acute effect of static stretching within a pre-event warm-up has received far more attention.

It was in the 1990s that more frequent investigations began into the role of stretching as part of a warm-up before training or competition. The common thought since the 1960s was that static stretching would improve performance, and Worrell and colleagues in 1994 (6) did report that four hamstring stretches of 15–20 seconds each improved eccentric and concentric leg flexion torque, as expected! As mentioned previously, the acute increase in range of motion (ROM) was thought to reduce resistance to movement, and to provide greater limb excursions which would be important for work output (work = force × linear or angular distance), running stride length, activities that need substantial flexibility (e.g. gymnastics, dance, figure skating, and others), and other movements. The proposition that improved flexibility would improve performance arises from the concepts of stress, strain, stiffness, and the modulus of elasticity. Stress and strain are related because they are defined as either the applied force divided by the tissue cross-sectional area (stress) or the ratio or change in tissue length with an applied force (strain). Stress and strain are directly related to tissue stiffness because stiffness is defined as the ratio of stress to strain or the ratio of changes in force to changes in length. Often the term "compliance" is used as the opposite to stiffness. A more compliant muscle or tendon is a less stiff muscle or tendon. Historically, Robert Hooke found that there was a proportional relationship between force and elongation. According to his modulus of elasticity, stiffer tissues need a greater stress (force or load) to produce a greater strain (change in length). Thus, a more compliant or less stiff musculotendinous unit should need less force or load to move it through a ROM, resulting in a greater economy of movement, and less resistance to movement.

But Kokkonen and colleagues in 1998 were among the first to contradict the prevailing notion that increased flexibility would improve performance. They found that five stretches involving six repetitions of 15 seconds each decreased knee flexion and extension force by 7–8% (7). A 1999 study by Avela et al. (8) had participants receive 1 hour of repeated passive static stretching, reporting impairments in force, electromyography (EMG), and reflex sensitivity. Typical of the problem with many of these earlier studies is the real-world relevance. What percentage of the population stretches their calf muscles for 60 minutes?

This led to many more studies in the early part of the millennium reporting stretching-induced impairments. A number of comprehensive reviews have reported that prolonged static stretching can lead to subsequent impairments in strength, power, sprint speed, agility, balance, evoked contractile properties, and other performance and physiological parameters (9–12). These impairments, on average range, from 4% to 7.5%. Static stretching can even impair the extent of muscle hypertrophy, strength, and insulin-like growth factor-1 (IGF-1) (13) achieved if you consistently stretch before or during resistance training. These reports have led to changes in how athletes prepare or warm up for training and competition. Whereas static stretching was widespread before the new millennium, there has been a shift away from static stretching to more dynamic stretching and dynamic activities. A review of American college tennis coaches in a 2012 article showed that 87% of coaches always employed a warm-up and, within that warm-up, 38.5% used a combination of static and dynamic stretching, 10.5% used only static stretching, and the rest relied primarily on dynamic activities and dynamic stretching (14). The results were slightly different for American university cross-country and track-and-field coaches in a 2013 article, with 98.1% always ensuring a warm-up, and within that group 44.7% used a combination of static and dynamic stretching, whereas 41.5% only performed dynamic stretching and 10.5% used static or proprioceptive neuromuscular facilitation (PNF) stretching (15). Their throwing counterparts used a warm-up 95.6% of the time, with 40.7% using dynamic stretching, 38.5% employing a combination of static and dynamic stretching, and 11.1% using static or PNF stretching (16). So, although the warm-up paradigm has shifted to an emphasis on dynamic stretching or a combination, about 10% of coaches in these studies still use static stretching alone. Is this paradigm shift a legitimate movement based on irrefutable fact or one of the many fads that we see come and go over the decades?

With static stretching-induced impairments, the emphasis should be placed on the term "prolonged" static stretching. It is generally agreed that ≥60 seconds of static stretching per muscle group is more likely to cause significant performance decrements (9–11). Muscle length is also a mitigating factor. Static stretches performed at short muscle lengths showed substantially greater deficits (10.2%), whereas static stretching at long muscle lengths actually resulted in small strength gains (2.2%) (9).

PNF stretching results from our review (11 PNF studies) which reported approximately 4% performance deficits (9). An earlier review (2007) found no clear evidence for a negative effect of PNF stretching on subsequent exercise performance (17). Sarah Marek and colleagues found that both static and PNF stretching led to similar strength, power, and muscle activation impairments, but the magnitude of the deficits were small (18). Therefore, as usual, there is never complete agreement in science. There are actually some studies that show PNF-induced improvements in isokinetic torque (6) and postural stability (19). But contradicting these studies are others reporting either no changes in strength or jump height (20) or PNF-induced deficits in proprioception (21), movement time, hip flexion angular velocity (22), vertical jump height (23,24), strength, power, and muscle activation (18). One study showed that 10 repetitions of PNF stretching increased blood lactate concentration, indicating there would be a greater reliance on anaerobic metabolism after PNF stretching (25). In the few studies that compared static and PNF stretching, PNF presented greater (6.4% vs 2.3%) subsequent deficits than the static stretching protocols. An important note to keep in mind is that most of these studies intervened only with prolonged stretching, without the additional activity you typically experience in a warm-up. The methodological problems and misinterpretations of these types of studies are examined later. But if you use only static or PNF stretch and do not have time to commit to a full warm-up procedure, how important are the consequences?

Although a 5% deficit (10) might not seem that dramatic to the average athlete, it can be devastating to an élite athlete. Usain Bolt won the 100-metre gold medal at the 2012 Olympic Games in 9.63 seconds. If a competitor were 5% slower, then where would he place in the competition? In fact, Gerard Phiri from Zambia was almost exactly 5% slower and ran the 100 metres in 10. 11 seconds. Did Phiri medal? Did Phiri make it to the finals? No, Gerard Phiri came in second last place (15th) in the semi-finals. The 5% difference was devastating. Usain Bolt makes millions of dollars from competing and endorsements, and I can bet that 99.9% of the readers have never heard of Gerard Phiri. Adidas, Nike, or Reebok is not knocking at his door, throwing money at him. Perhaps you watched the 2016 Olympics and saw Bolt win again in 9.81 seconds (he was getting older and slowed down!). As a Canadian, I was cheering for Andre De Grasse, who won a bronze medal in 9.91 seconds (Figure 8.1). The difference between Bolt and De Grasse was 1.009%. Performing the correct warm-up is unbelievably crucial in élite competitions. In our 2011 review (10) we stated:

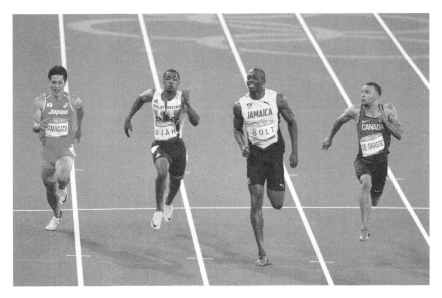

FIGURE 8.1 Olympic sprint 2016

It would be wise to be cautious when implementing static stretching of any duration or for any population when high-speed, rapid stretch-shortening cycle, explosive or reactive forces are necessary, particularly if any decreases in performance, however small, would be important.

(p 264)

However, there are a number of caveats to this statement. We also mentioned that (p 9): "All individuals should include static stretching in their overall fitness and wellness activities for the health and functional benefits associated with increased ROM and musculotendinous compliance". In our 2016 review (9), which involved a more expansive and critical examination of the literature, we modified our views and said the following:

When a typical pre-event warm-up is complete (i.e. initial aerobic activity, stretching component, 5–15 min of task- or activity-specific dynamic activities), the benefits of SS and PNF stretching for augmented ROM and reduced injury risk balance, or may outweigh, any possible cost of (trivial) performance decrements.

Sounds very confusing! Should we stretch or not before explosive or high-speed training or competition?

To simplify the answer, it might be easier to think of yourself either as a Ferrari or a Cadillac (Figure 8.2). Élite athletes are the Ferrari, Lamborghini, or Bugati sports cars of the world. The purpose of the élite athlete is to push

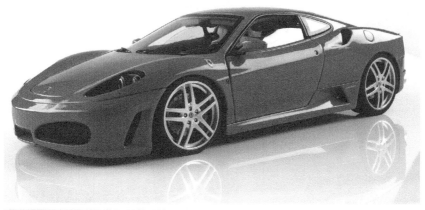

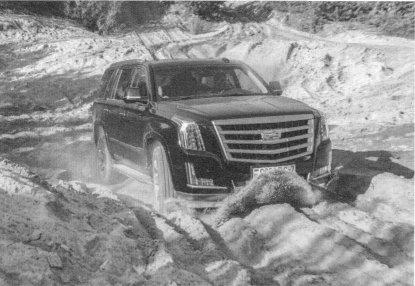

FIGURE 8.2 Ferrari (tighter suspension) versus Cadillac (more compliant, less stiff suspension)

themselves to their physiological, anatomical, and psychological limits. They need to produce maximal forces, or power; many times in the briefest possible periods they exert extremely high pressures, torques, impacts, and other stresses to their body. Usain Bolt and the other international calibre sprinters have foot contact times on the track of less than 100 ms. Thus, they must hit the ground and take off without absorbing and losing much energy. Élite sprinters will leave the starting blocks in about 120–160 ms (26). The fastest start was by Bruny Surin (another Canadian) at 101 ms in the 1999 world championship semi-final. Athletes with stiffer or less compliant musculotendinous systems are reported to be more economical runners (less energy expended for the same amount of work) than their more flexible counterparts (27–29). A number of studies have reported that static stretching can reduce sprinting speed (30–35). Similar to human sprinters, a Ferrari sports car needs to accelerate from the start and move out of curves and corners rapidly. To accomplish this task, sports cars have tight suspension so they react to the road immediately. Driving a Ferrari over a bumpy road would not be much fun and in fact excruciatingly painful for your lower back because the suspension would not absorb much of the shock of the potholes in the roads. For the average city or country road, you want a car with nice soft suspension that absorbs the shocks, so that the driver feels almost nothing when encountering a bump in the road. A Cadillac and other similar cars have great suspensions that effectively absorb these shocks. You would never expect a Cadillac to beat a Ferrari in a race, especially on a route that included curves and turns. After every race, mechanics must examine, repair, or replace the damaged components of sports cars. There are always damaged parts after every race. The car has been pushed to its mechanical limit and the suspension did not adequately absorb or reduce the effect of the road environment on the other parts of the Ferrari. You would understandably be very upset if, every time you drove your Cadillac, you had to bring it to the mechanic to get it repaired. The top sprinters (Bolt and colleagues), tennis players (Federer, Djokovic, and colleagues), and other individual sports athletes, as well as team sports athletes, have athletic trainers, physiotherapists, massage therapists, and others ready to provide them with treatment immediately after a competition when they have pushed their bodies to the limit. The average fitness enthusiast and weekend warrior athlete does not have a cadre of health practitioners to treat him or her after every workout. Most of the population do not push themselves to the extreme limit.

There is no single correct prescription for the optimal degree of flexibility. Everybody has their "Goldilocks" zone. The élite sprinter needs to transfer contractile forces as quickly as possible from the muscle to the tendon to the bone, resulting in movement. If a tendon is overly slack (high compliance) there will be a negative impact on electromechanical delay (EMD). The EMD is the time it takes for the muscle to be activated, contract, pull, and tighten the tendon and then have the bone move. Under laboratory conditions the EMD is measured as the duration between the onset of the muscle action potential wave (M-wave) and the onset of force or torque production (Figure 8.3). If an élite athlete's parallel (muscle membranes) and series elastic (i.e. tendons) components were very compliant, then the EMD would be prolonged and the time it takes for a muscle contraction to actually result in movement would also be lengthened. This of course is anathema to the élite sprinter who wants to explode out of the blocks in the shortest time (reaction time) or spend the least amount of time in contact with the track (increased stride rate).

Previously, I told you that prolonged static stretching or increased flexibility can decrease running economy. However, there are also studies that contradict these previous studies with reports that static stretching also decreased the energy cost of

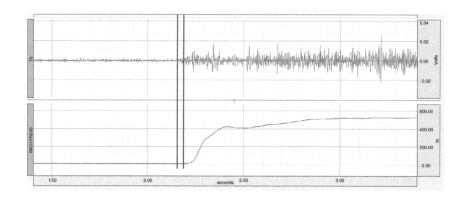

**Evoked
EMD**

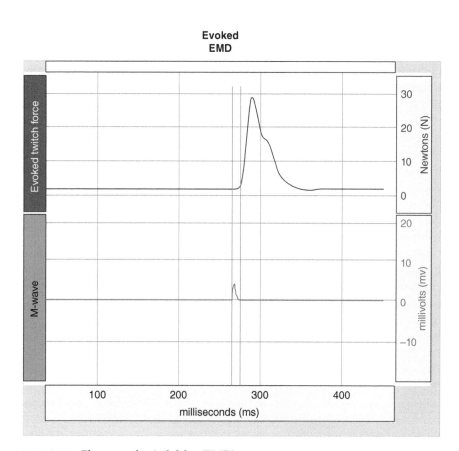

FIGURE 8.3 Electromechanical delay (EMD)

running (36) or had no effect (37). How is this possible? Were one set of scientists incompetent and incorrect? No, it is necessary to look at the specificity of the task. Schmidtbleicher (38) defined two types of rebound jumps or stretch-shortening cycle (SSC) actions (Figures 8.4 and 8.5). A jump performed with a contact time of <250 ms was classified as a short SSC and >250 ms was considered a long SSC. The two studies that found improved running economy with prior stretching used submaximal, slower, prolonged running (i.e. 40%, 60%, or 80% of maximum O_2 consumption or below lactate threshold) with long SSC. With slower running and longer SSC, the person is in longer contact with the ground (Figure 8.6). A very stiff musculotendinous system absorbs the reaction forces over a very short period and returns the energy to the muscles very quickly (desirable for sprinters). If the system is very stiff, the mechanical and reflex energy return (SSC) would occur while the slower runner is still in the landing phase and not ready to propel him- or herself into the next stride. A more compliant or flexible muscle and tendon would absorb the reaction forces over a longer period, and the spring-like action of the muscles and tendons would return the energy to the muscles when the distance runner is ready to push off the ground.

Studies that examine evoked contractile properties (electrical stimulation of the muscle or nerve) might give some insight into some of the mechanisms underlying static stretch-induced impairments. A few studies have reported static stretch-induced decreases in twitch force, rate of force development, and prolonged EMD (39–42). As a reminder, EMD is primarily affected by the musculotendinous unit (MTU) compliance or stiffness. It has been suggested that there is a direct relationship between EMD and muscle stiffness (43). If the MTU is more compliant, it will take longer to transfer the energy of the myofilament cross-bridge kinetics to the muscle and tendon tissues to move the bone. Muscle stiffness has a greater influence on athletic performance than flexibility (44). The intrinsic or baseline stiffness of a muscle can still be

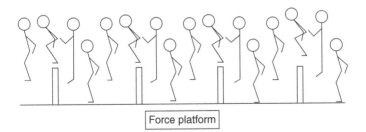

Force platform

FIGURE 8.4 Stretch-shortening cycle: hurdle jumps (from right to left) beginning with take-off (propulsion), flight phase, (clearance of the hurdle), landing (involving eccentric contractions to absorb the reaction forces), with a short contact (amortization or transition phase) time, followed by concentric contractions for another propulsion phase

moderately high and yet, with a high tolerance to stretch (pain or discomfort), an individual can still have substantial levels of flexibility.

Some researchers have compared a mechanomyogram (MMG) signal with the force or EMG signal to parcel out the EMD associated with excitation–contraction coupling and MTU viscoelastic properties. An MMG monitors changes in the muscle shape by sensing vibrations and oscillations of the muscle fibres at the resonant frequency of the muscle. With a higher signal-to-noise ratio than the surface EMG, it is purported to be able to monitor muscle activity from deeper muscles. After five sets of 45 seconds of passive stretching, the excitation–contraction (E-C) coupling aspect of the EMD (Δt: EMG–MMG) was prolonged for approximately 15 minutes, whereas the MTU viscoelasticity (Δt: MMG–tetanic force) was

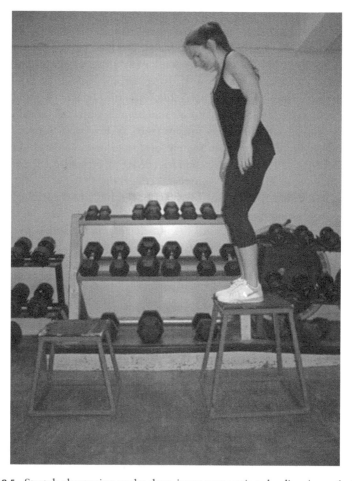

FIGURE 8.5 Stretch-shortening cycle: drop-jump preparation, landing (amortization or transition phase with elongation/stretching of muscles and tendons), and take-off (propulsion: concentric contractions)

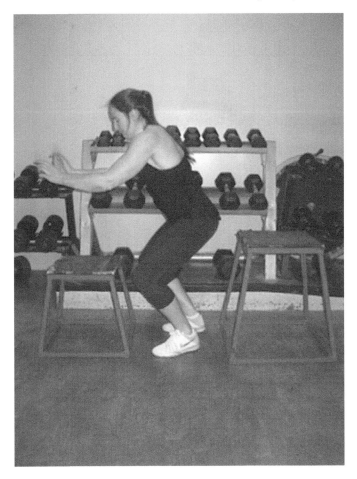

FIGURE 8.5   (Cont.)

prolonged for up to 2 hours (45). It is necessary to remind the reader that research is almost never unanimous. A study from our lab also found force deficits up to 2 hours after stretching two muscles for three sets of 45 seconds each. However, although there were significant voluntary force deficits (10%), the evoked twitch and tetanic force deficits (1–4%) were non-significant over that same period (46). However, peak tetanic force has also been reported to be depressed for 2 hours after five repetitions of 45-second static stretches with 15 seconds of rest between stretches (41). Changes in evoked twitch forces represent changes in E-C coupling (muscle action potential leading to the release and sequestration of calcium from the sarcoplasmic reticulum) and tetanic forces represent changes in myofilament kinetics. Hence, five repeats of 45 seconds of stretching in this one study damaged the myosin and actin cross-bridges, which would affect not only peak force but also probably the rate of force development.

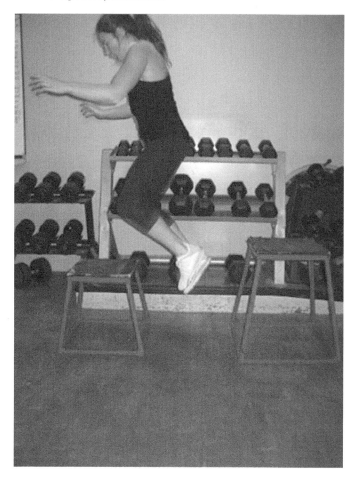

FIGURE 8.5 (Cont.)

The Goldilocks flexibility or ROM zone for sprinters versus distance runners would be different based on their differing ground contact times. Further evidence for task specificity of stretching is provided by experiments that demonstrated a 5% increase in a rebound chest press (5) and no significant effects on an isometric bench press (47). As the amortization or transition phase from the eccentric to the concentric phases of a bench press would be much slower than the contact time during sprinting, a more compliant system would be able to absorb and return the elastic energy in a more appropriate task-specific time period.

Effects of static stretching on the stretch-shortening cycle

The SSC is an important neuromuscular mechanism that enhances power production with rapid, explosive activities and contractions. Prime examples of

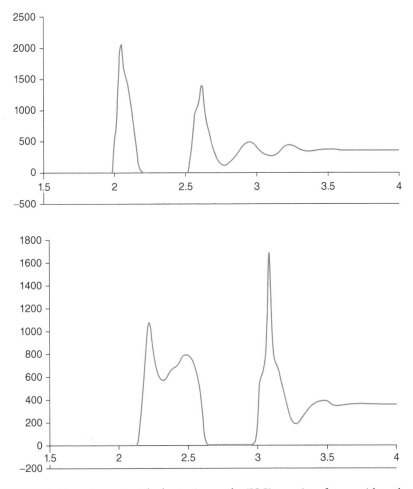

FIGURE 8.6 Drop-jump stretch-shortening cycle (SSC) reaction forces with a short versus long contact time

SSC activities are plyometric activities such as counter-movement, hurdle and drop jumps, hopping, bounding, skipping, sprinting, and other similar activities. With SSC activities, external forces (e.g. body mass accelerated by gravity) lengthen the muscle during an active contraction (eccentric phase), which is followed by a concentric (shortening) contraction (48,49). SSC exercises use the elastic energy that was stored during the eccentric contraction phase to augment the concentric phase (50,51). This augmentation involves both mechanical (musculotendinous) and neural (reflexive) components. Similar to an elastic band, the contractile elements (i.e. myosin) and muscle connective tissue (i.e. titin, desmin) and tendons are stretched, resulting in the storage of potential elastic energy, which is returned to the neuromuscular system shortly thereafter.

The energy stored in the system can be extremely high. For example, a study from our laboratory reported that hurdle jumps that emphasized short contact times generated mean reaction forces of 4335 newtons (442 kg or 972 lb). This reaction force was approximately 5.5 times the body mass and approximately 100% higher than the much slower SSC action of counter-movement jumps (52). The elongation of the MTU does not need to be extensive to achieve this elastic rebound. A tendon elongation of 6–7% during the stretching phase is sufficient to elicit the SSC. Rack and Westbury (53) originally labelled this small elongation short-range elastic stiffness. If the tendon can return elastic energy with only a 6–7% elongation, we can see why sprinters may not need or want a very compliant MTU. A stiffer MTU is still fine for transferring elastic recoil energy.

The duration for the return of this elastic recoil depends on the compliance or elasticity of the SSC. A tighter system will return this elastic recoil earlier than a more compliant system. Slow SSC actions get only a minor contribution from the passive elastic elements, creating a greater reliance on muscle contractile properties to produce concentric phase force. However, a rapid SSC can take greater advantage of elastic energy from the MTU (54,55). With rapid SSC actions, the cross-bridges can remain attached during the stretch, to augment the force during the concentric phase (56). The rapid deceleration during the eccentric stretch phase, followed by the acceleration during the propulsive, concentric phase, contributes to a power potentiation and improved energy economy that depend on the speed of the eccentric stretch phase (55).

Not only is there a mechanical elastic storage and energy return but also the SSC causes an excitation of the muscle spindle reflexes (57). Rapid SSC actions induce greater reaction forces, muscle reflex activity, and muscle activation (58). The muscle spindles sense and react to changes in the extent and rate of muscle lengthening. Within the muscle spindle, nuclear chain fibres preferentially respond to changes in the amount of stretch or elongation of the muscle, whereas the nuclear bag fibres respond to both the extent of elongation and the rate. These signals return to the spinal motoneurons via annulospiral (high conduction velocity) and flower-spray endings (low conduction velocity) through Ia (nuclear bag and chains) and II (nuclear chains) afferents, respectively. A monosynaptic myotactic reflex is initiated from the rapid stretch action, resulting in the depolarization/activation (contraction) of the α-motoneuron of the stretched muscle and inhibition (disynaptic) of the antagonist muscle (59). This reflex action aids in neural potentiation, stiffening the contractile components due to the myofilament cross-bridge attachments, and augmenting the active contraction forces.

The spindle afferents can contribute up to 30% to the activation of the motoneurons (60). Persistent inward currents (PICs) from previous contractions contribute to motoneuron depolarization during the subsequent contractions. PICs are a depolarizing inward current of motoneurons that respond to brief synaptic input with prolonged firing activity, even after the input stops (known as self-sustained firing). They can also increase the maximum motoneuron firing rate. PICs are derived from Na^+ and low-voltage-activated L-type Ca^{2+} ion channels. A small afferent signal that activates the dendritic PIC is amplified, creating a larger current to the soma (motoneuronal body), which produces higher motoneuronal firing rates (61). It is interesting that neurophysiologists use the term "warm-up" for the increased activation of the Ca^{2+} PIC. Thus, the increased reflex afferent activity from repeated SSC actions, in concert with supraspinal drive, would potentiate the motoneuron response (i.e. greater rate coding). However, a number of static stretching studies have reported Hoffmann (H)-reflex (afferent excitability of the spinal motoneuron) inhibition with stretching (8,62–65). Thus, static stretching could inhibit this neural potentiation.

There are many explosive, power-type athletes such as gymnasts and figure skaters who have extensive flexibility and yet still have a rapid and efficient SSC. Does this not contradict the previous discussion? These types of athletes can perform powerfully even with a very compliant MTU if they actively stiffen the system before contracting. Hence, it is important for them to pre-activate the system. More experienced and accomplished athletes will pre-activate the muscles with a feed-forward (pre-planned) central command (66). The first 40 ms of ground contact time is too soon for spindle reflexes to stiffen the system, and thus pre-activation from supraspinal activation is necessary (67).

Static stretching effects on balance

There is some evidence that improved dorsiflexion ROM can facilitate balance test performance (anterior direction in the Star Excursion Balance Test or SEBT) (68) and, even with 10–30 minutes of static or dynamic stretching (15-second repetitions) with a 5-minute aerobic warm-up, there was a small magnitude improvement in SEBT performance (69). The SEBT is usually performed under controlled and slower conditions, and thus a less stiff, more compliant system that reacts over a more prolonged period could provide better feedback and postural adjustments for this test. The improved SEBT performance with greater flexibility might not necessarily translate to the far more rapid adjustments to posture (metastability) encountered with such high-velocity perturbations found with downhill skiing, rugby, American football, and other sports or everyday activities such as slipping on an icy sidewalk. Although proprioception can affect balance, another study using 3×30 seconds of static stretching showed no effect of stretching on knee position sense (proprioception) (70).

Effects of flexibility training

Are the effects of stretching mitigated by population age, gender, trained state, or other considerations? Perhaps the reason that so many studies report static stretch-induced deficits is due to the fact that most people do not stretch on a regular basis. If we took a group of untrained people and had them resistance train or go for a long run, they would certainly be sore and weak for days afterwards.

Untrained people would experience deficits even with mild-to-moderate strength or aerobic training. So, would people who train for stretching regularly not experience these stretch-induced deficits? A study from our laboratory reported that 5 weeks of stretch training improved ROM by 12–20%, but the participants still experienced deficits of 6–8% in leg strength and jump height (71). In the same study, we tested a diverse group of people and ranked them by their flexibility. We thought that perhaps the most flexible people might not be as adversely affected by prolonged static stretching. We performed a cross-sectional correlation and did not find any significant relationship between hip and ankle ROM and static stretch-induced deficits in force and jump height. Furthermore, the Behm and Chaouachi review (10) examined 41 stretching studies with trained individuals versus 68 studies using untrained individuals. They did not find any significant difference overall between the two groups, with both experiencing stretch-induced deficits. Prolonged static stretching shows no favourites: trained and untrained, flexible or inflexible people are still susceptible to the adverse effects.

Ageing effects

There are very few studies examining the effects of stretching on middle-aged and older populations. The reports are contradictory, with some studies reporting no impairments (72) and others showing impairments (73). Thus, it seems that, although the results from individual studies can be contradictory, in general all segments of the population from young to old may experience static stretch-induced impairments from prolonged static stretching that is not accompanied by the dynamic active components of a full warm-up.

Effect of stretching intensity

The literature emphasizes the importance of stretch duration for determining whether performance deficits will be incurred (9–11). These reviews agree that fewer than 60 seconds of static stretching per muscle group should be implemented if static stretch-induced impairments are to be minimized. What about the intensity of stretching? If some individual stretches to the point of maximal discomfort or pain is it more likely to lead to performance deficits than if they performed lower intensity stretching? Is it "more pain, less gain" for performance after stretching? Once again, the answer is not clear. There are some studies showing no impairments when the stretch was held to a point of "mild" discomfort (74–77), which are contradicted by others that do show performance decrements with stretching to a point of mild discomfort (23,33,78–80). In a study from our laboratory, participants stretched quadriceps, the hamstrings. and plantar flexors for three repetitions of 30 seconds each either to100%, 75%, or 50% of the point of maximal discomfort. All stretching intensities adversely affected jump height. To be cautious, individuals should expect performance deficits if they stretch at any intensity for more than 60 seconds per muscle group, without the inclusion of any other dynamic activity within the warm-up.

Cost–benefit analysis

To consider how much flexibility is needed by an individual, a subjective cost–benefit analysis should be conducted. The possible **cost** of prolonged static stretching without a full warm-up is performance impairments of 4–8%. The possible **benefits** of static stretching are a greater ROM, more shock absorption, and lower incidence of musculotendinous injuries. A stiff musculotendinous system does not absorb forces well and is more susceptible to strains and sprains. Furthermore, how much ROM is necessary to achieve your goals? As a sprinter, soccer rugby, or ice hockey player, and others, a moderate degree of flexibility is necessary. A gymnast, dancer, figure skater, competitive diver, ice hockey goalie, and others need more extreme ROM. To the vast majority of the population who are recreationally active, the cost of possible minor impairments pales in comparison to the cost of injury. A reasonable individual would probably surmise that hitting the golf ball 10 yards or meters shorter is a reasonable price to pay to ensure that he or she can continue playing golf multiple times a week throughout the season without injury.

Effects of dynamic stretching on performance

In contrast to static and PNF stretching, dynamic stretching is reported to produce (mean of 48 studies) trivial to small (1.3%) performance enhancements (9). The Canadian Society for Exercise Physiology position stand and meta-analysis illustrated that dynamic stretching improved performance in 20 studies (small or greater than small effect sizes), and showed trivial effects in 21 studies and impairments in 7 studies (9). Measures included counter-movement jumps, sprints, agility, isometric and isokinetic force, or torque and power, 1RM (1 repetition maximum), balance, and other variables. The average reader should always be cognizant that, even when a textbook or a review reports overall significant or meaningful improvements or impairments, a close inspection of the individual studies in the literature almost always shows a spectrum of results that are influenced by the protocol, subject/participant population, type of measures, or other variables. Thus, general summaries or recommendations can be made on the global review of the literature, but there is always the possibility for each individual that their response to a stressor such as stretching might not behave similarly to the grand aggregate means reported in these books and reviews.

The review by Behm and Chaouachi (10) recommended that more than 90 seconds of dynamic stretching should be performed for each muscle group; however, the studies are quite variable in their durations, so a dose–response relationship for dynamic stretching is more difficult to establish (9). In these studies, the durations of dynamic stretching can range from 1 minute to

20 minutes with either some performance enhancement or no adverse effects. Similarly, there seems to be a tendency for performance improvements with faster dynamic stretches or more intense ballistic stretches, but there is a high degree of variability in the literature, so definitive statements about dynamic stretching duration or frequency (speed) also cannot be made at this time. So, if dynamic activities and stretching tend to excite the central nervous system whereas static stretching tends to depress it, would a combination of dynamic and static stretching within a warm-up counterbalance each other?

Effects of combining static and dynamic stretching on performance

As reported earlier, the studies by Judge and colleagues reported that 39–45% of American college coaches for tennis, and track and field, use a combination of static and dynamic stretching in their warm-up. Unfortunately, real-world practices are not paralleled by the volume of research in this area. Thus, even with the scant research combining dynamic and static stretching, can we say whether the neural excitation of the dynamic stretching counteracts the neural inhibition/disfacilitation of the static stretching? Not always! The research results vary from impairments to no change to improvements. In one study, the combination of static and dynamic stretching resulted in 50-metre sprint time impairments compared with dynamic stretching alone (32). Another study showed no difference and no vertical jump impairments when comparing dynamic stretching with a combination of static and dynamic stretching (81). However, maybe Gaelic footballers are unique because in a study using Irish athletes, 20- and 40-metre sprint speed (0.7–1.0%) and counter-movement jump height (8.7%) improved with a combination of static and dynamic stretching (82). A study from our lab, used four conditions: (1) general aerobic warm-up with static stretching; (2) general aerobic warm-up with dynamic stretching; (3) general and sport-specific warm-up with static stretching; and (4) general and sport-specific warm-up with dynamic stretching. We found that, when a sport-specific warm-up was included, there was a 1% improvement ($P = 0.001$) in 20-metre sprint time with both the dynamic and the static stretch groups. Without a sport-specific warm-up, there were no such improvements. In addition, static stretching increased sit-and-reach (hamstrings and lower back) ROM approximately 3% more than the dynamic stretching. In another study, the combination of static and dynamic stretching was not detrimental for the agility of professional soccer players, but dynamic stretching was more effective for preparing for agility (83).

Is performance affected if the individual stretches between sets of a resistance-training workout? A study that compared heavy load-resistance training (3 sets × 4 repetitions) with heavy load-resistance training with stretching (3 × 15 seconds) between sets reported no effect of interset stretching on jump height (84).

As the research recommends fewer than 60 seconds of static stretching per muscle group, so as not to induce impairments, and that many of the ROM studies favour static stretching over dynamic stretching for the greatest ROM increases, it would seem reasonable to recommend a combination of brief (<60 seconds) static stretching with >90 seconds per muscle group of dynamic stretching, in addition to a previous >5 minutes of aerobic activity, and a subsequent 5–15 minutes of activity-specific dynamic activity, to ensure an optimal ROM with either no deficits or perhaps even enhancement of performance. This type of warm-up has been reported in the literature to increase ROM without subsequent impairments or, in some cases, actually to improve some aspects of performance (9).

Effects of ballistic stretching on performance

Ballistic and dynamic stretching are often confused as being the same action. As mentioned earlier, dynamic stretching involves moving a joint actively through a full ROM under controlled conditions (not maximum speed), whereas ballistic stretching is usually performed at higher speeds, often with bouncing movements at the end of the ROM. As usual, the literature is not unanimous. Some articles report that ballistic stretching has no significant effect on subsequent strength (85,86), vertical jump height (23,87), or plantar flexors'-passive–resistive torque (88), whereas others report impairments in knee flexion and extension strength (89,90), fatigue endurance (86,89), passive–resistive torque, and muscle (91) and Achilles tendon stiffness (88). On the other hand, Fletcher used the term "fast dynamic stretching" for movements at 100 beats/min, which might be considered ballistic. With these fast dynamic (possibly ballistic) stretches, they found an increase in vertical jump height and EMG compared with slow dynamic stretches or no stretching at all. In all these studies, a full warm-up (initial aerobic component, static stretching, or slow dynamic stretching followed by sport-specific dynamic activity) was not incorporated. Hence, these cited studies should warn us about performing ballistic stretches as the only activity in a warm-up because there is the definite possibility for performance decrements. The next section describes the problems of interpreting such delimited studies when applying their results to the real world.

Full warm-ups

The emphasis in the previous section was to warn about the negative effects of "prolonged" static and PNF stretching. The typical stretch durations for professional basketball, American football, ice hockey, and baseball players ranges from 12 seconds to 17 seconds (92–95). However, in the research you see stretch durations of 9–13 repetitions of 135 s each (20–30 min for the plantar flexors) (40,96). One of our early studies had participants perform 20 minutes of quadriceps stretching (97). Scientists would say that these studies lack "ecological validity", i.e. they are not representative of what actually happens in the real world. Almost nobody would stretch one muscle group for 20–30 minutes, especially without all the components of a full warm-up before a training session or competition. Many of the static stretching studies in the literature lack ecological validity (real-world application). As you would imagine most of these prolonged static stretching studies had substantial stretch-induced deficits.

Another major problem is that most studies intervened with a stretching-only protocol with no or little other dynamic activity (9). The traditional or conventional pre-activity warm-up protocol consists of an initial submaximal or low-intensity exercise component (e.g. running, cycling) that increases the heart rate and muscle temperature (remember the effects of heat on ROM), as well as exciting/activating the neuromuscular system. This aerobic segment is followed by static stretching, which according to our recommendations should not exceed more than 60 seconds per muscle group (9–11). Dynamic stretching should also be involved to provide more task- and velocity-specific ROM-augmenting activity. The final aspect involves activity or sport-specific dynamic activity that further activates the cardiovascular, neuromuscular, endocrine, and other physiological systems in preparation for the activity (9,98). The few studies that do include a full warm-up typically do not illustrate significant stretch-inducing deficits or may provide some performance improvements (99–103). One of our collaborative studies demonstrated that the combination of previous running, followed by static stretching, finishing with counter-movement jumps resulted in 7–17% better jump performances versus static stretching alone (104). In another collaborative study with our colleagues in Tunisia, the combination of static and dynamic stretching at different static stretching intensities (point of discomfort and less than point of discomfort) resulted in no significant impairments. Thus, the inhibition or depression of the neuromuscular system with prolonged static stretching seems to be balanced by the excitation of the system with dynamic warm-up activities.

A recent fairly definitive study by our lab (105) has demonstrated relatively clearly the interaction of static stretch duration and the dynamic components of the warm-up. In this study, participants went through a full warm-up protocol including a 5-minute aerobic warm-up, followed by a static stretching component, dynamic stretching component, and finally a sport-specific dynamic activity component. They either did static stretches of 30, 60, or 120 seconds or no static stretching within this warm-up protocol. Participants were tested after each component as well as 10 minutes after the warm-up. All conditions improved hamstrings and quadriceps ROM. There were no impairments in maximal voluntary contraction (MVC) forces, jump height with the control, and 30 seconds of static stretching at any time. Impairments were evident with 120 seconds of stretching for quadriceps force (post-static stretching and at 10 minutes after warm-up), force produced in the first 100 ms (post-static stretching), and muscle activation (10 minutes post-warm-up). Vertical jump improved with the warm-up activities except for 60 and 120 seconds of static stretching, when tested immediately after the static stretching component. Thus, as the Behm et al. review (9) proposed, static stretching of <60 seconds per muscle group within a full warm-up should not lead to performance impairments. The lack of static stretch-induced impairments when incorporated within a full warm-up could be due to the post-activation potentiation effect of the dynamic activities. Kummel et al. (106) reported the typical static stretch deficits but, when they added hops, there was no difference from the control condition although the jump heights were significantly higher than with the stretch-only condition. Similarly, 10 minutes of dynamic stretching were sufficient to potentiate vertical jump characteristics (107). Even adding a deadlift did not augment the potentiating effect on vertical jump. Thus, dynamic stretching alone can potentiate performance and offset possible impairments from prolonged static stretching.

These findings were also substantiated by Blazevich and colleagues (108) who incorporated 30 seconds of static stretching into a full warm-up, and reported increased ROM but no impairments in jumping, sprinting, or agility tests. A very interesting aspect of their study was that they asked the participants about their performance expectations when stretching was included. Before the study, 18/20 participants nominated dynamic stretching as the most likely to improve performance and 15/20 participants nominated no stretching to be least likely. None the less, these ratings were not related to test performances. The authors suggested that including static or dynamic stretching into a warm-up routine instilled more confidence in the participants with regard to their performance in the ensuing sports-related tests. As psychological effects are so potent for optimal performance, and appropriate durations of static and dynamic stretching generally do not seem to degrade performance when incorporated into a full warm-up (Table 8.1), it might be a good idea to include short-to-moderate durations of static stretching (<60 seconds) into a complete warm-up.

Improving performance by limiting muscle soreness

Excessive unaccustomed activity, especially those activities that emphasize eccentric contractions, can lead to exercise-induced muscle damage (EIMD) and lead to delayed-onset muscle soreness (DOMS) which can persist for 5–7 days (109,110). EIMD and DOMS can decrease force, power, running speed, neuromuscular efficiency (extent of muscle activation needed to accomplish a task), ROM, and many other performance factors (111–113). It has been a common belief that stretching can either prevent or reduce EIMD and DOMS. Stretching before, during, or after the EIMD-induced exercise did not reduce subsequent DOMS (110,114–116). A review by Howatson and van Someren (117) also concluded that stretching to prevent or reduce EIMD provides only minimal effects in reducing muscle soreness with no performance effects. Some early studies reported that, during DOMS, static stretch-induced reductions in muscle activity (measured with EMG or measurement of the H-reflex to muscle action potential ratio) (118–121) contributed to reduced soreness. For a similar reason (decreased muscle activity) (120,122), static stretching tends to relieve muscle cramps (123–125). Other possible suggested mechanisms for DOMS

TABLE 8.1 Full warm-up components

Submaximal aerobic activity	Static stretching	Dynamic stretching	Task-specific activities
5–15 minutes of running, cycling or other activity to increase muscle temperatures, decrease tissue viscoelasticity, and increase heart rate, enzymatic cycling, and other factors	<60 seconds per muscle group No need to go to the point of discomfort or pain Stretch major muscle groups and specific muscle groups to the activity	>90 seconds per muscle group Use full ROM with a controlled movement at moderate speeds.	5–15 minutes Practise movements that are associated with the sport or task at velocities close to the actual movement.

relief would be that stretching helps to remove some of the inflammation or swelling associated with DOMS (126). Furthermore, stretching during DOMS could initiate the gate control theory of pain suppression (127), whereby the activation of higher-velocity afferents (i.e. type Ia or Ib) from mechanical stimulation of stretch, cutaneous, and other receptors can inhibit the slower velocity pain afferents such as type IV afferents (128) (Figure 8.7). A common example of the gate control theory is the typical response to an injured finger, limb, or other body part. The immediate response is to grab that injured body part and start rubbing it. Rubbing the area activates the high-velocity, cutaneous, tactile or pressure receptors which help to block the slower afferents peripherally and centrally from the nociceptors (pain receptors). Typically, there is never just one mechanism and thus DOMS reduction could be a combination of a number of mechanisms.

Limitations of acute stretching studies

Another limitation of most stretch research studies is the post-stretch testing period. After the warm-up, do most athletes or teams immediately begin their competition? Many athletes or teams go back to their dressing room or bench to finalize tactics and strategies, make equipment adjustments, and other necessities (i.e. pre-game renal voiding). For some competitions, there is a national anthem to start the game. But the average time to testing after a warm-up was 3.2, 4.9, and 4.1 minutes for static, dynamic, and PNF stretching studies (9). Once again, the ecological validity can be questioned because many athletes would not start their competition less than 5 minutes after their warm-up.

Furthermore, who are the participants in these studies? As most of the studies are conducted at the kinesiology, physical education, sport, or exercise science departments of universities, the students are likely to be familiar with these studies that report stretch-induced impairments. A study from our laboratory tried to

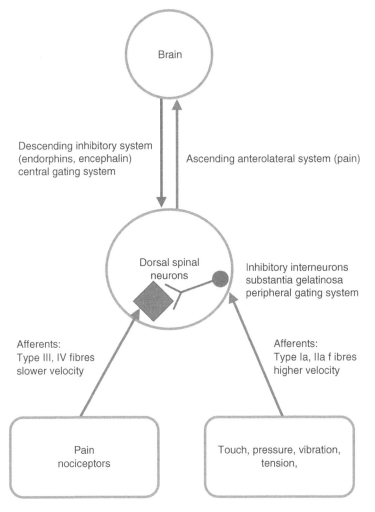

FIGURE 8.7   Gate control theory of pain (127)

deceive the participants by telling non-kinesiology students that stretching would actually improve their performance and compared their responses with those of kinesiology students (knowledgeable about the stretching literature) after three static hamstrings stretches of 30 seconds each. Both groups still experienced hamstring force and activation deficits due to stretching, but the deceived group experienced improvements in the performance of the antagonist quadriceps muscle. Therefore, the deception could not overcome the stretching impairments of the hamstrings (90 seconds was 50% more than the recommended ≤60 seconds) but quadriceps, which was not stretched, was susceptible to the deception that stretching would improve performance. Hence, bias and deception could play a small role in these types of studies. Furthermore, there is bias in the journal publications for studies that provide significant findings (129). For example, it is more difficult to publish a study that reports no changes with stretching than one that would report significant decrements. Our review found that reporting of data/statistics within published papers was less common when non-significant results were obtained. In most studies the details of non-significant changes were commonly not reported, which could result in an overestimation of the stretching deficit effects (9).

Summary

Throughout the second half of the twentieth century, it was commonly believed that static stretching-induced increases in muscle compliance (reduced stiffness) would enhance subsequent performance by allowing a greater ROM with less resistance to movement. However, static and PNF stretching studies from the late 1990s into the early 2000s predominantly reported subsequent performance impairments of 3–7.5%. These findings changed the traditional warm-up paradigm, shifting the emphasis from static to dynamic stretching within a warm-up. Specifically, it was found that prolonged static stretching (>60 seconds per muscle group) without all components of a full warm-up increased the chances of performance deficits. The decision to include static stretching within a warm-up may depend on the type or demands of the activity (i.e. jogging with minimal ROM needs versus hurdling with increased flexibility needs), the level of the athlete (élite vs recreational), and the priority of reducing the incidence of musculotendinous injuries compared with the possible 3–4% performance decrements. Prolonged static stretching without a full warm-up can impair performance in both trained and untrained individuals, young and old, whether the stretch is performed at a moderate or a high intensity.

Dynamic stretching, on the other hand, may have either no significant impairments or actually provide small enhancements of subsequent performance. Adding static to dynamic stretching tends to counterbalance possible impairments with prolonged static stretching. Individuals should incorporate at least 90 seconds of dynamic stretching per muscle group within a full warm-up. The full warm-up should include a 5- to 15-minute submaximal aerobic component, <60 seconds of static stretching per muscle group, >90 seconds of dynamic stretching per muscle group, and finish with dynamic activity that should be activity or sport specific.

References

1. Dintiman GB. Effects of various training programs on running speed. *Res Q* 35: 456–463, 1964.
2. Nelson AG, Kokkonen J, Eldredge C, Cornwell A, and Glickman-Weiss E. Chronic stretching and running economy. *Scand J Med Sci Sports* 11: 260–265, 2001.
3. Yuktasir B and Kaya F. Investigation into the long term effects of static and PNF stretching exercises on range of motion and jump preformance. *J Bodyw Mov Ther* 13: 11–21, 2009.

4. Bazett-Jones DM, Gibson MH, and McBride JM. Sprint and vertical jump performances are not affected by six weeks of static hamstring stretching. *J Strength Cond Res* 22: 25–31, 2008.

5. Wilson G, Elliot B, and Wood G. Stretching shorten cycle performance enhancement through flexibility training. *Med Sci Sports Exerc* 24: 116–123, 1992.

6. Worrell T, Smith T, and Winegardner J. Effect of hamstring stretching on hamstring muscle performance. *J Orthop Sports Phys Ther* 20: 154–159, 1994.

7. Kokkonen J, Nelson AG, and Cornwell A. Acute muscle stretching inhibits maximal strength performance. *Res Q Exerc Sport* 69: 411–415, 1998.

8. Avela J, Kyrīlñinen H, and Komi PV. Altered reflex sensitivity after repeated and prolonged passive muscle stretching. *J Appl Physiol* 86: 1283–1291, 1999.

9. Behm DG, Blazevich AJ, Kay AD, and McHugh M. Acute effects of muscle stretching on physical performance, range of motion, and injury incidence in healthy active individuals: A systematic review. *Appl Physiol Nutr Metab* 41: 1–11, 2016.

10. Behm DG and Chaouachi A. A review of the acute effects of static and dynamic stretching on performance. *Eur J Appl Physiol* 111: 2633–2651, 2011.

11. Kay AD and Blazevich AJ. Effect of acute static stretch on maximal muscle performance: A systematic review. *Med Sci Sports Exerc* 44: 154–164, 2012.

12. Shrier I. Does stretching improve performance?: A systematic and critical review of the literature 39. *Clin J Sport Med* 14: 267–273, 2004.

13. Borges Bastos CL, Miranda H, Vale RG, Portal Mde N, Gomes MT, Novaes Jda S, and Winchester JB. Chronic effect of static stretching on strength performance and basal serum IGF-1 levels. *J Strength Cond Res* 27: 2465–2472, 2013.

14. Judge LW, Bellar D, Craig B, Petersen J, Camerota J, Wanless E, and Bodey K. An examination of preactivity and postactivity flexibility practices of National Collegiate Athletic Association Division I tennis coaches. *J Strength Cond Res* 26: 184–191, 2012.

15. Judge LW, Petersen JC, Bellar DM, Craig BW, Wanless EA, Benner M, and Simon LS. An examination of preactivity and postactivity stretching practices of crosscountry and track and field distance coaches. *J Strength Cond Res* 27: 2456–2464, 2013.

16. Judge LW, Bellar DM, Gilreath EL, Petersen JC, Craig BW, Popp JK, Hindawi OS, and Simon LS. An examination of preactivity and postactivity stretching practices of NCAA division I, NCAA division II, and NCAA division III track and field throws programs. *J Strength Cond Res* 27: 2691–2699, 2013.

17. Rubini EC, Costa AL, and Gomes PS. The effects of stretching on strength performance. *Sports Med* 37: 213–224, 2007.

18. Marek SM, Cramer JT, Fincher AL, Massey LL, Dangelmaier SM, Purkayastha S, Fitz KA, and Culbertson JY. Acute effects of static and proprioceptive neuromuscular facilitation stretching on muscle strength and power output. *J Athl Train* 40: 94–103, 2005.

19. Ryan EE, Rossi MD, and Lopez R. The effects of the contract–relax-antagonist–contract form of proprioceptive neuromuscular facilitation stretching on postural stability. *J Strength Cond Res/Natl Strength Cond Assoc* 24: 1888–1894, 2010.

20. Young W and Elliott S. Acute effects on static stretching, proprioceptive neuromuscular facilitation stretching, and maximum voluntary contractions on explosive force production and jumping performance. *Res Q Exerc Sport* 72: 273–279, 2001.

21. Streepey JW, Mock MJ, Riskowski JL, Vanwye WR, Vitvitskiy BM, and Mikesky AE. Effects of quadriceps and hamstrings proprioceptive neuromuscular facilitation stretching on knee movement sensation. *J Strength Cond Res* 24: 1037–1042, 2010.

22. Maddigan ME, Peach AA, and Behm DG. A comparison of assisted and unassisted proprioceptive neuromuscular facilitation techniques and static stretching. *J Strength Cond Res/Natl Strength Cond Assoc* 26: 1238–1244, 2012.

23. Bradley PS, Olsen PD, and Portas MD. The effect of static, ballistic, and proprioceptive neuromuscular facilitation stretching on vertical jump performance. *J Strength Cond Res* 21: 223–226, 2007.

24. Church JB, Wiggins MS, Moode EM, and Crist R. Effect of warm-up and flexibility treatments on vertical jump performance. *J Strength Cond Res* 15: 332–336, 2001.

25. Gultekin Z, Kin-Isler A, and Surenkok O. Hemodynamic and lactic acid responses to proprioceptive neuromuscular facilitation excercise. *J Sports Sci Med* 5: 375–380, 2006.

26. Mero A and Komi PV. Reaction time and electromyographic activity during a sprint start. *Eur J Appl Physiol Occup Physiol* 61: 73–80, 1990.

27. Gleim GW, Stachenfeld NS, and Nicholas JA. The influence of flexibility on the economy of walking and jogging. *J Orthop Res* 8: 814–823, 1990.

28. Jones AM. Running economy is negatively related to sit-and-reach test performance in international-standard distance runners. *Int J Sports Med* 23: 40–43, 2002.

29. Trehearn TL and Buresh RJ. Sit-and-reach flexibility and running economy of men and women collegiate distance runners. *J Strength Cond Res* 23: 158–162, 2009.

30. Beckett JR, Schneiker KT, Wallman KE, Dawson BT, and Guelfi KJ. Effects of static stretching on repeated sprint and change of direction performance. *Med Sci Sports Exerc* 41: 444–450, 2009.

31. Chaouachi A, Chamari K, Wong P, Castagna C, Chaouachi M, Moussa-Chamari I, and Behm DG. Stretch and sprint training reduces stretch-induced sprint performance deficits in 13- to 15-year-old youth. *Eur J Appl Physiol* 104: 515–522, 2008.

32. Fletcher IM and Anness R. The acute effects of combined static and dynamic stretch protocols on fifty-meter sprint performance in track-and-field athletes. *J Strength Cond Res* 21: 784–787, 2007.

33. Sayers AL, Farley RS, Fuller DK, Jubenville CB, and Caputo JL. The effect of static stretching on phases of sprint performance in elite soccer players. *J Strength Cond Res* 22: 1416–1421, 2008.

34. Siatras T, Papadopoulos G, Mameletzi DN, Vasilios G, and Kellis S. Static and dynamic acute stretching efect on gymnasts' speed in vaulting. *Pediatric Exerc Sci* 15: 383–391, 2003.

35. Winchester JB, Nelson AG, Landin D, Young MA, and Schexnayder IC. Static stretching impairs sprint performance in collegiate track and field athletes. *J Strength Cond Res* 22: 13–19, 2008.

36. Godges JJ, MacRae H, Longdon C, and Tinberg C. The effects of two stretching procedures on the economy of walking and jogging. *J Orthop Sport Phys Ther* 7: 350–357, 1989.

37. Hayes PR and Walker A. Pre-exercise stretching does not impact upon running economy. *J Strength Cond Res* 21: 1227–1232, 2007.

38. Schmidtbleicher D. Training for power events. In: *Strength and power in sport.* Komi PV, ed. Oxford: Blackwell Publishers, 1992, pp 381–395.

39. Ce E, Paracchino E, and Esposito F. Electrical and mechanical response of skeletal muscle to electrical stimulation after acute passive stretching in humans: A combined electromyographic and mechanomyographic approach. *J Sports Sci* 26: 1567–1577, 2008.

40. Costa PB, Ryan ED, Herda TJ, Walter AA, Hoge KM, and Cramer JT. Acute effects of passive stretching on the electromechanical delay and evoked twitch properties. *Eur J Appl Physiol Occup Physiol* 108: 301–310, 2010.

41. Esposito F, Limonta E, and Ce E. Passive stretching effects on electromechanical delay and time course of recovery in human skeletal muscle: New insights from an electromyographic and mechanomyographic combined approach. *Eur J Appl Physiol* 111: 485–495, 2011.

42. Ryan ED, Beck TW, Herda TJ, Hull HR, Hartman MJ, Stout JR, and Cramer JT. Do practical durations of stretching alter muscle strength? A dose–response study. *Med Sci Sports Exerc* 40: 1529–1537, 2008.

43. Grosset JF, Piscione J, Lambertz D, and Perot C. Paired changes in electromechanical delay and musculo-tendinous stiffness after endurance or plyometric training. *Eur J Appl Physiol Occup Physiol* 105: 131–139, 2009.

44. Rey E, Padron-Cabo A, Barcala-Furelos R, and Mecias-Calvo M. Effect of high and low flexibility levels on physical fitness and neuromuscular properties in professional soccer players. *Int J Sports Med* 37: 878–883, 2016.

45. Esposito F, Ce E, Rampichini S, and Veicsteinas A. Acute passive stretching in a previously fatigued muscle: electrical and mechanical response during tetanic stimulation. *J Sports Sci* 27: 1347–1357, 2009.

46. Power K, Behm D, Cahill F, Carroll M, and Young W. An acute bout of static stretching: effects on force and jumping performance. *Med Sci Sports Exerc* 36: 1389–1396, 2004.

47. Torres EM, Kraemer WJ, Vingren JL, Volek JS, Hatfield DL, Spiering BA, Ho JY, Fragala MS, Thomas GA, Anderson JM, Hakkinen K, and Maresh CM. Effects of stretching on upper body muscular performance. *J Strength Cond Res* 22: 1279–1285, 2008.

48. Komi PV. *The stretch-shortening cycle and human power output*. Champaign, IL: Human Kinetics, 1986.

49. Norman RW and Komi PV. Electromechanical delay in skeletal muscle under normal movement conditions. *Acta Physiol\Scand* 106: 241–248, 1979.

50. Cavagna GA, Dusman B, and Margaria R. Positive work done by a previously stretched muscle. *J Appl Physiol* 24: 21–32, 1968.

51. Komi PV and Bosco C. Utilization of stored elastic energy in leg extensor muscles by men and women. *Med Sci Sports* 10: 261–265, 1978.

52. Cappa DF and Behm DG. Training specificity of hurdle vs. countermovement jump training. *J Strength Cond Res/Natl Strength Cond Assoc* 25: 2715–27202011.

53. Rack PM and Westbury DR. The short range stiffness of active mammalian muscle and its effect on mechanical properties. *J Physiol* 240: 331–350, 1974.

54. Cronin J, McNair PJ, and Marshall RN. Power absorption and production during slow, large-amplitude stretch-shorten cycle motions. *Eur J Appl Physiol* 87: 59–65, 2002.

55. Ishikawa M, Komi PV, Finni T, and Kuitunen S. Contribution of the tendinous tissue to force enhancement during stretch-shortening cycle exercise depends on the prestretch and concentric phase intensities. *J Electromyogr Kinesiol* 16: 423–431, 2006.

56. Baptista RR, Scheeren EM, Macintosh BR, and Vaz MA. Low-frequency fatigue at maximal and submaximal muscle contractions. *Braz J Med Biol Res* 42: 380–385, 2009.

57. Nicol C and Komi PV. Significance of passively induced stretch reflexes on Achilles tendon force enhancement. *Muscle Nerve* 21: 1546–1548, 1998.

58. Toumi H, Poumarat G, Best TM, Martin A, Fairclough J, and Benjamin M. Fatigue and muscle-tendon stiffness after stretch-shortening cycle and isometric exercise. *Appl Physiol Nutr Metab* 31: 565–572, 2006.

59. McArdle WD, Katch FI, and Katch VL. *Exercise physiology: Energy, nutrition, and human performance*. Malvern, PA: Lea & Febiger, 1991.

60. Gandevia SC. Neural control in human muscle fatigue: changes in muscle afferents, moto neurones and moto cortical drive. *Acta Physiol Scand* 162: 275–283, 1998.

61. ElBasiouny SM, Schuster JE, and Heckman CJ. Persistent inward currents in spinal motoneurons: Important for normal function but potentially harmful after spinal cord injury and in amyotrophic lateral sclerosis. *Clin Neurophysiol* 121: 1669–1679, 2010.

62. Etnyre BR and Abraham LD. H-reflex changes during static stretching and two variations of proprioceptive neuromuscular facilitation techniques. *Electroencephalogr Clin Neurophysiol* 63: 174–179, 2005.

63. Guissard N and Duchateau J. Neural aspects of muscle stretching. *Exerc Sport Sci Rev* 34: 154–158, 2006.

64. Guissard N, Duchateau J, and Hainaut K. Muscle stretching and motoneuron excitability. *Eur J Appl Physiol* 58: 47–52, 1988.

65. Guissard N, Duchateau J, and Hainaut K. Mechanisms of decreased motoneurone excitation during passive muscle stretching. *Exp Brain Res* 137: 163–169, 2001.

66. Dietz V, Schmidtblecher D, and Noth J. Neuronal mechanisms of human locomotion. *J Neurophysiol* 42: 1212–1222, 1979.

67. Gollhofer A, Strojnik V, Rapp W, and Schweizer L. Behaviour of triceps surae muscle–tendon complex in different jump conditions. *Eur J Appl Physiol Occup Physiol* 64: 283–291, 1992.

68. Hoch MC, Staton GS, and McKeon PO. Dorsiflexion range of motion significantly influences dynamic balance. *J Sci Med Sport* 14: 90–92, 2011.

69. Belkhiria-Turki L, Chaouachi A, Turki O, Hammami R, Chtara M, Amri M, Drinkwater EJ, and Behm DG. Greater volumes of static and dynamic stretching within a warm-up do not impair star excursion balance performance. *J Sports Med Phys Fitness* 54: 279–288, 2014.

70. Larsen R, Lund H, Christensen R, Rogind H, Danneskiold-Samsoe B, and Bliddal H. Effect of static stretching of quadriceps and hamstring muscles on knee joint position sense. *Br J Sports Med* 39: 43–46, 2005.

71. Behm DG, Bradbury EE, Haynes AT, Hodder JN, Leonard AM, and Paddock NR. Flexibility is not related to stretch-induced deficits in force or power. *J Sports Sci Med* 5: 33–42, 2006.

72. Handrakis JP, Southard VN, Abreu JM, Aloisa M, Doyen MR, Echevarria LM, Hwang H, Samuels C, Venegas SA, and Douris PC. Static stretching does not impair performance in active middle-aged adults. *J Strength Cond Res* 24: 825–830, 2010.

73. Behm DG, Plewe S, Grage P, Rabbani A, Beigi HT, Byrne JM, and Button DC. Relative static stretch-induced impairments and dynamic stretch-induced enhancements are similar in young and middle-aged men. *Appl Physiol Nutr Metab* 36: 790–797, 2011.

74. Knudson D, Bennett K, Corn R, Leick D, and Smith C. Acute effects of stretching are not evident in the kinematics of the vertical jump. *J Strength Cond Res* 15: 98–101, 2001.

75. Knudson DV, Noffal GJ, Bahamonde RE, Bauer JA, and Blackwell JR. Stretching has no effect on tennis serve performance. *J Strength Cond Res* 18: 654–656, 2004.

76. Manoel ME, Harris-Love MO, Danoff JV, and Miller TA. Acute effects of static, dynamic, and proprioceptive neuromuscular facilitation stretching on muscle power in women. *J Strength Cond Res* 22: 1528–1534, 2008.

77. Young W, Elias G, and Power J. Effects of static stretching volume and intensity on plantar flexor explosive force production and range of motion. *J Sports Med Phys Fitness* 46: 403–411, 2006.

78. Cramer JT, Housh TJ, Johnson GO, Miller JM, Coburn JW, and Beck TW. Acute effects of static stretching on peak torque in women. *J Strength Cond Res* 18: 236–241, 2004.

79. Cramer JT, Housh TJ, Weir JP, Johnson GO, Coburn JW, and Beck TW. The acute effects of static stretching on peak torque, mean power output, electromyography, and mechanomyography. *Eur J Appl Physiol* 93: 530–539, 2005.

80. Hough PA, Ross EZ, and Howatson G. Effects of dynamic and static stretching on vertical jump performance and electromyographic activity. *J Strength Cond Res* 23: 507–512, 2009.

81. Wallman HW, Mercer JA, and McWhorter JW. Surface electromyographic assessment of the effect of static stretching of the gastrocnemius on vertical jump performance. *J Strength Cond Res* 19: 684–688, 2005.

82. Loughran M, Glasgow P, Bleakley C, and McVeigh J. The effects of a combined static-dynamic stretching protocol on athletic performance in elite Gaelic footballers: a randomised controlled crossover trial. *Phys Ther Sport* 25: 47–54, 2017.

83. Khorasani MA, Sahebozamani M, Tabrizi KG, and Yusof AB. Acute effect of different stretching methods on illinois agility test in soccer players. *J Strength Cond Res* 24: 1–7, 2010.

84. Gonzalez-Rave JM, Machado L, Navarro-Valdivielso F, and Vilas-Boas JP. Acute effects of heavy-load exercises, stretching exercises, and heavy-load plus stretching exercises on squat jump and countermovement jump performance. *J Strength Cond Res* 23: 472–479, 2009.

85. Bacurau RF, Monteiro GA, Ugrinowitsch C, Tricoli V, Cabral LF, and Aoki MS. Acute effect of a ballistic and a static stretching exercise bout on flexibility and maximal strength. *J Strength Cond Res* 23: 304–308, 2009.

86. Barroso R, Tricoli V, Santos Gil SD, Ugrinowitsch C, and Roschel H. Maximal strength, number of repetitions, and total volume are differently affected by static-, ballistic-, and proprioceptive neuromuscular facilitation stretching. *J Strength Cond Res* 26: 2432–2437, 2012.

87. Jaggers JR, Swank AM, Frost KL, and Lee CD. The acute effects of dynamic and ballistic stretching on vertical jump height, force, and power. *J Strength Cond Res* 22: 1844–1849, 2008.

88. Mahieu NN, McNair P, De MM, Stevens V, Blanckaert I, Smits N, and Witvrouw E. Effect of static and ballistic stretching on the muscle-tendon tissue properties. *Med Sci Sports Exerc* 39: 494–501, 2007.

89. Lima CD, Brown LE, Wong MA, Leyva WD, Pinto RS, Cadore EL, and Ruas CV. Acute effects of static vs. ballistic stretching on strength and muscular fatigue between ballet dancers and resistance-trained women. *J Strength Cond Res* 30: 3220–3227, 2016.

90. Nelson AG and Kokkonen J. Acute ballistic muscle stretching inhibits maximal strength performance. *Res Q Exerc Sport* 72: 415–419, 2001.

91. Konrad A, Stafilidis S, and Tilp M. Effects of acute static, ballistic, and PNF stretching exercise on the muscle and tendon tissue properties. *Scand J Med Sci Sports* 27: 1070–1080, 2017.

92. Ebben WP and Blackard DO. Strength and conditioning practices of National Football League strength and conditioning coaches. *J Strength Cond Res* 15: 48–58, 2001.

93. Ebben WP, Carroll RM, and Simenz CJ. Strength and conditioning practices of National Hockey League strength and conditioning coaches. *J Strength Cond Res* 18: 889–897, 2004.

94. Ebben WP, Hintz MJ, and Simenz CJ. Strength and conditioning practices of Major League Baseball strength and conditioning coaches. *J Strength Cond Res* 19: 538–546, 2005.

95. Simenz CJ, Dugan CA, and Ebben WP. Strength and conditioning practices of National Basketball Association strength and conditioning coaches. *J Strength Cond Res* 19: 495–504, 2005.

96. Fowles JR, Sale DG, and MacDougall JD. Reduced strength after passive stretch of the human plantar flexors. *J Appl Physiol* 89: 1179–1188, 2000.

97. Behm DG, Button DC, and Butt JC. Factors affecting force loss with prolonged stretching. *Can J Appl Physiol* 26: 261–272, 2001.

98. Young W and Behm D. Should static stretching be used during a warm-up for strength and power activities? *J Strength Cond* 24: 33–37, 2002.

99. Little T and Williams AG. Effects of differential stretching protocols during warm-ups on high-speed motor capacities in professional soccer players. *J Strength Cond Res* 20: 203–207, 2006.

100. Murphy JR, Di Santo MC, Alkanani T, and Behm DG. Aerobic activity before and following short-duration static stretching improves range of motion and performance vs. a traditional warm-up. *Appl Physiol Nutr Metab* 35: 679–690, 2010.

101. Samson M, Button DC, Chaouachi A, and Behm DG. Effects of dynamic and static stretching within general and activity specific warm-up protocols. *J Sports Sci Med* 11: 279–285, 2012.

102. Taylor JM, Weston M, and Portas MD. The effect of a short practical warm-up protocol on repeated sprint performance. *J Strength Cond Res* 27: 2034–2038, 2013.

103. Wallmann HW, Mercer JA, and Landers MR. Surface electromyographic assessment of the effect of dynamic activity and dynamic activity with static stretching of the gastrocnemius on vertical jump performance. *J Strength Cond Res* 22: 787–793, 2008.

104. Young WB and Behm DG. Effects of running, static stretching and practice jumps on explosive force production and jumping performance. *J Sports Med Phys Fitness* 43: 21–27, 2003.

105. Reid JC, Greene R, Young JD, Hodgson DD, Blazevich AJ, and Behm DG. The effects of different durations of static stretching within a comprehensive warm-up on voluntary and evoked contractile properties. *Eur J Appl Physiol*, 118 (7): 1427–1445, 2018.

106. Kummel J, Kramer A, Cronin NJ, and Gruber M. Postactivation potentiation can counteract declines in force and power that occur after stretching. *Scand J Med Sci Sports*, 27 (12): 1750–1760, 2016.

107. Turki O, Chaouachi A, Drinkwater EJ, Chtara M, Chamari K, Amri M, and Behm DG. Ten minutes of dynamic stretching is sufficient to potentiate vertical jump performance characteristics. *J Strength Cond Res* 25: 2453–2463, 2011.

108. Blazevich AJ, Gill ND, Kvorning T, Kay AD, Goh A, Hilton B, Drinkwater EJ, and Behm DG. No effect of muscle stretching within a full, dynamic warm-up on athletic performance. *Med Sci Sports Exerc*, https://doi.org/10.1249/MSS.0000000000001539, 2018.

109. Behm DG, Baker KM, Kelland R, and Lomond J. The effect of muscle damage on strength and fatigue deficits. *J Strength Cond Res* 15: 255–263, 2001.

110. Gulick DT, Kimura IF, Sitler M, Paolone A, and Kelly JD. Various treatment techniques on signs and symptoms of delayed onset muscle soreness. *J Athl Train* 31: 145–152, 1996.

111. Byrnes WC and Clarkson PM. Delayed onset muscle soreness and training. *Clin Sports Med* 5: 605–615, 1986.

112. Cleak MJ and Eston RG. Delayed onset muscle soreness: Mechanisms and management. *J Sports Sci* 10: 325–341, 1992.
113. Connolly DA, Sayers SP, and McHugh MP. Treatment and prevention of delayed onset muscle soreness. *J Strength Cond Res* 17: 197–208, 2003.
114. Buroker KC and Schwane JA. Does postexercise static stretching alleviate delayed muscle soreness? *Phys Sportsmed* 17: 65–83, 1989.
115. Herbert RD and Gabriel M. Effects of stretching before and after exercising on muscle soreness and risk of injury: Systematic review. *BMJ* 325: 468, 2002.
116. High DM, Howley ET, and Franks BD. The effects of static stretching and warm-up on prevention of delayed-onset muscle soreness. *Res Q Exerc Sport* 60: 357–361, 1989.
117. Howatson G and Van Someren KA. The prevention and treatment of exercise-induced muscle damage. *Sports Med* 38: 483–503, 2008.
118. De Vries HA. Electromyographic observation of the effect of static stretching upon muscular distress. *Res Q* 4: 468–479, 1961.
119. De Vries HA. Prevention of muscular distress after exercise. *Res Q* 2: 177–185, 1961b.
120. De Vries HA. Quantitative electromyographic investigation of the spasm theory of muscle pain. *Am J Phys Med* 45: 119–134, 1966.
121. Thigpen LK, Moritani T, Thiebaud R, and Hargis JL. The acute effects of static stretching on alpha motoneuron excitability. In: *Biomechanics IX-A International Series on Biomechanics*. Winter DA, Norman RW, Wells RP, Hayes KC, and Patla AE, ed. Champaign, IL: Human Kinetics, 1985, pp 352–357.
122. Helin P. Physiotherapy and electromyography in muscle cramp. *Br J Sports Med* 19: 230–231, 1985.
123. Bertolasi L, De Grandis D, Bongiovanni LG, Zanette GP, and Gasperini M. The influence of muscular lengthening on cramps. *Ann Neurol* 33: 176–180, 1993.
124. Davison S. Standing: a good remedy. *JAMA* 252: 3367, 1984.
125. Weiner IH and Weiner HL. Nocturnal leg muscle cramps. *JAMA* 244: 2332–2333, 1980.
126. Bobbert MF, Hollander AP, and Huijing PA. Factors in delayed onset muscular soreness of man. *Med Sci Sports Exerc* 18: 75–81, 1986.
127. Melzack R and Wall PD. Pain mechanisms: a new theory. *Science* 150: 971–979, 1965.
128. Armstrong RB. Mechanisms of exercise-induced delayed onset muscular soreness: a brief review. *Med Sci Sports Exerc* 16: 529–538, 1984.
129. Easterbrook PJ, Berlin JA, Gopalan R, and Matthews DR. Publication bias in clinical research. *Lancet* 337: 867–872, 1991.

9

EFFECT OF STRETCH TRAINING ON PERFORMANCE

Static stretching

Although acute prolonged static stretching can lead to impairments, there are physiological rationales why chronic static stretching could improve performance. Static stretch training can enhance Ca^{2+} within the neuromuscular junction (1), decrease muscle stiffness (2), and proliferate sarcomeres in series (3,4). Increased neuromuscular junction Ca^{2+} should enhance neurotransmitter release. Decreased musculotendinous stiffness or increased compliance could reduce the resistance to movement, improving movement and energy efficiency. Energy efficiency would be directly related to a training-related decrease in hysteresis (5), which is related to tissue viscoelastic changes affecting heat loss with stretching (6). Thus training-induced changes in viscoelasticity leading to decreased hysteresis (the return to the original state is delayed) would help retain rather than dissipate energy through heat loss (5). Furthermore, increased musculotendinous unit compliance could positively affect the stretch-shortening cycle (SSC) by enhancing the ability to store elastic energy (2,5). This compliance-induced elastic storage enhancement would be more apparent with longer-duration eccentric-to-concentric transitions such as a rebound chest press (2), but might not have such a positive impact on very short SSC activities such as sprinting where the athlete might transition from foot strike to take-off in less than 100 ms.

A higher number of sarcomeres in series could allow muscle to produce more force or torque at longer muscle lengths and change the optimal force angle (7). It has been reported that many of the musculotendinous injuries occur at extended muscle lengths, when the muscle exerts lower forces and cannot protect itself, to a great extent, as well against environmental stressors (8). Another advantage is that the number of sarcomeres in series is related to muscle contraction velocity

(9). As a reminder, however, increases in sarcomere number with stretching have been primarily verified in animal studies but not human in vivo studies.

A well-cited review by Shrier (10) reported that regular stretching would improve most athletic performances. Another systematic review (5) showed that only half of the stretch-training articles (14/28) improved muscle performance. There was very little effect on static or isometric contraction measures. Muscle performance improvements in these studies were generally dynamic activities such as jumps, isokinetic eccentric and concentric torque, rebound bench press, and plantar flexors 1RM (1 repetition maximum). However, even with dynamic activities the results were not consistent. Similar to the Behm et al. (8) review, which suggested a major advantage of stretching would be enhanced force outputs at longer muscle lengths, the Medeiros and Lima review (5) found a number of studies reporting enhanced eccentric peak torque. As eccentric contractions are ubiquitous in all activities, but especially important in SSC activities because they help to potentiate or augment the concentric contraction (11,12), a flexibility training-induced improvement in eccentric strength could be of vital importance. As you should suspect by now, none of these statements ever gets unanimous support. A 6-week stretch-training study incorporating either static or proprioceptive neuromuscular facilitation (PNF) stretching showed similar improvements in range of motion (ROM) but no effect on drop-jump performance (13). Another 6-week static stretch-training programme with female track-and-field athletes did not improve knee ROM, or sprint or vertical jump performance (14). A strength-training study that incorporated static stretching before each workout, before each set, or no stretching reported that, although all groups improved strength over the 10-week training period, the no-stretch group had greater muscle strength and IGF-1 (insulin-like growth factor) improvements.

Dynamic stretch training

When dynamic stretching was incorporated into the daily warm-up of wrestlers for 4 weeks there were improvements in power, strength, muscular endurance, anaerobic capacity, and agility performance (15). Similarly, an 8-week pro-gramme involving either active (not staying in one spot) or static (staying in one location) dynamic stretch training improved both flexibility and jump parameters but not sprint performance (16).

Summary

In contrast to the reported performance impairments with acute bouts of prolonged static stretching, there are many physiological adaptations with static stretch training that should enhance performance. However, the evidence from static stretch-training studies is contradictory. The few dynamic stretch studies that there are do show performance improvements but not with every measure.

References

1. Yamashita T, Ishii S, and Oota I. Effect of muscle stretching on the activity of neuromuscular transmission. *Med Sci Sports Exerc* 24: 80–84, 1992.
2. Wilson G, Elliot B, and Wood G. Stretching shorten cycle performance enhancement through flexibility training. *Med Sci Sports Exer* 24: 116–123, 1992.
3. De Deyne PG. Application of passive stretch and its implications for muscle fibers. *Phys Ther* 81: 819–827, 2001.
4. Zollner AM, Abilez OJ, Bol M, and Kuhl E. Stretching skeletal muscle: Chronic muscle lengthening through sarcomerogenesis. *PLoS One* 7: e45661, 2012.
5. Medeiros DM and Lima CS. Influence of chronic stretching on muscle performance: Systematic review. *Hum Mov Sci* 54: 220–229, 2017.
6. Kubo K. In vivo elastic properties of human tendon structures in lower limb. *Int J Sport Health Sci* 3: 143–151, 2005.
7. Chen TC, Lin KY, Chen HL, Lin MJ, and Nosaka K. Comparison in eccentric exercise-induced muscle damage among four limb muscles. *Eur J Appl Physiol* 111: 211–223, 2011.
8. Behm DG, Blazevich AJ, Kay AD, and McHugh M. Acute effects of muscle stretching on physical performance, range of motion, and injury incidence in healthy active individuals: a systematic review. *Appl Physiol Nutr Metab* 41: 1–11, 2016.
9. Lieber RL and Bodine-Fowler SC. Skeletal muscle mechanics: Implications for rehabilitation. *Phys Ther* 73: 844–856, 1993.
10. Shrier I. Does stretching improve performance? A systematic and critical review of the literature 39. *Clin J Sport Med* 14: 267–273, 2004.
11. Cappa DF and Behm DG. Training specificity of hurdle vs. countermovement jump training. *J Strength Cond Res/Natl Strength Cond Assoc* 25: 2715–2720, 2011.
12. Cappa DF and Behm DG. Neuromuscular characteristics of drop and hurdle jumps with different types of landings. *J Strength Cond Res* 27: 3011–3020, 2013.
13. Yuktasir B and Kaya F. Investigation into the long term effects of static and PNF stretching exercises on range of motion and jump preformance. *J Bodyw Mov Ther* 13: 11–21, 2009.
14. Bazett-Jones DM, Gibson MH, and McBride JM. Sprint and vertical jump performances are not affected by six weeks of static hamstring stretching. *J Strength Cond Res* 22: 25–31, 2008.
15. Herman SL and Smith DT. Four-week dynamic stretching warm-up intervention elicits longer-term performance benefits. *J Strength Cond Res* 22: 1286–1297, 2008.
16. Turki-Belkhiria L, Chaouachi A, Turki O, Chtourou H, Chtara M, Chamari K, Amri M, and Behm DG. Eight weeks of dynamic stretching during warm-ups improves jump power but not repeated or single sprint performance. *Eur J Sport Sci* 14: 19–27, 2014.

10

OTHER FLEXIBILITY-ENHANCING TECHNIQUES

Massage, foam rolling, and roller massage

Stretching is not the only technique that can be used to enhance range of motion (ROM). Massage has been used since recorded history as a relaxation technique, cure for specific illnesses, and performance enhancer. The first written records of the use of massage originated in Egypt and China. A Chinese text entitled *The Yellow Emperor's Classic Book of Internal Medicine* was written around 2700 BCE. Egyptian tomb paintings around 2500 BCE illustrate massage as a medical therapy while written records of massage in India originate from 1500 BCE to 500 BCE. Western civilizations did not use massage as medical or health therapy until Per Ling from Sweden incorporated hand stroking into the Swedish Movement System in the early 1800s. Recently, devices such as foam rollers and roller massagers have become quite popular as self-massage therapy (Figure 10.1) (1–7).

Originally, these devices were branded as "self-myofascial release" devices that could aid in reducing (myo)fascial restrictions. Fascial restrictions are reported to occur in response to injury, disease, inactivity, and inflammation. Purportedly, if fascia loses its elasticity and becomes dehydrated, fascia or connective tissue can bind around the traumatized areas, causing formation of a fibrous adhesion (8,9). These myofascial adhesions may create "hypersensitive tender spots" (10), also known as trigger points. Fibrous adhesions can be painful, prevent normal muscle mechanics (i.e. neuromuscular hypertonicity, and decreased strength, endurance, and motor coordination), and decrease soft-tissue extensibility, negatively affecting joint ROM and muscle length (8,9).

Rolling involves small undulations back and forth over the affected muscle with a dense foam roller, typically starting at the proximal portion of the muscle,

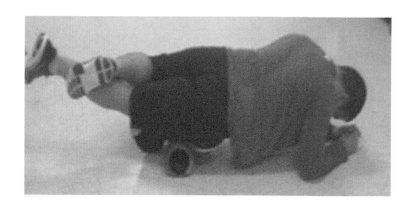

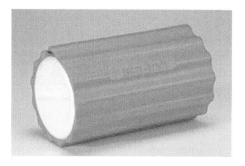

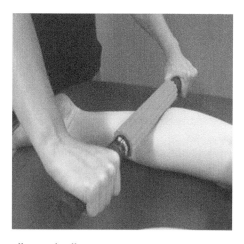

FIGURE 10.1 Foam rollers and roller massagers

working down to the distal portion of the muscle, or vice versa. Foam rollers are quite diverse in their composition, with some made from poly(vinyl chloride) pipe surrounded by neoprene foam, whereas others may be made from closed cell foam. Roller massagers are typically composed of dense foam wrapping around a solid plastic cylinder. There are many variations, with some having a ridged design that is supposed to allow for both superficial and deep-tissue massage (2,7). The most recent modification is to have vibrating rollers.

Rolling has been shown to acutely increase ROM (1–7,11) with changes continuing for as long as 20 minutes (12–14). ROM increases are highly variable ranging from 3% to 23% (11,15). One of the major concerns about prolonged static stretching was the evidence for subsequent performance impairments (16,17). One of the advantages of rolling is that, although it can increase ROM, it does not typically affect subsequent athletic performance (18). These performance measures have included measures of muscle strength, power, and balance (3,5,7,19–21).

So how does rolling increase ROM? One of the more obvious mechanisms is thixotropy. As discussed in Chapter 4, thixotropic effects occur when viscous (thicker) fluids become less viscous or more fluid like when agitated, sheared, or stressed. When the stress is removed, or desists, then the fluid takes a certain period to return to the original viscous state. The rolling undulations place direct and sweeping pressure on the soft tissues, generating friction. The increased friction-related temperature of the soft tissues and the stress from the rolling can decrease the viscosity of intracellular and extracellular fluids, providing less resistance to movement. Remember the cold car and oil analogy.

The use of the term self-myofascial release suggests that rolling will help to release myofascial adhesions, allowing freer, less restricted movement. However, it is suggested that the amount of force needed to remove adhesions would exceed the physiological limitations of most people (8,9). Partial body mass on a foam roller or the force applied on a roller massager with the arms would be insufficient to break up these adhesions. So, do rollers only work through thixotropy?

Golgi tendon organs (GTOs – type Ib afferents) respond to musculotendinous tension and strong stretch, usually resulting in inhibition. A study from our laboratory (22) demonstrated that using a single bout of a short-duration (10- or 30-second) massage at the hamstring musculotendinous junction increased ROM with no increase in passive muscle tension or electromyographic (EMG) activity: 30 seconds of musculotendinous massage provided greater overall ROM than 10 seconds. Although one might assume that the tension applied to the tendon would activate the inhibitory responses of the GTOs, leading to greater muscle relaxation or decreased tonus, the GTO effects persist for only about 60 ms after cessation of stress (23). Thus, the respective 5.8–11.3% ROM increases immediately after the massage could not be due to GTO inhibition.

Muscle, fascia, and skin are densely innervated by sensory neurons (8,9). Within the epidermis and dermis (skin layers), there are mechanoreceptors such as Merkel's receptors, Meissner's corpuscles, Ruffini's cylinders, and Pacinian corpuscles, which have different sized receptor fields, adapt slowly or rapidly, and respond to different frequencies of skin stimulation. Merkel's discs (small receptor field) and Ruffini's cylinders (large receptor field) are slowly adapting and respond as long as the stimulus is present, whereas Meissner's (small receptor field) and pacinian (large receptor field) corpuscles are rapidly adapting and thus respond to stimulation with a burst of firing activity at the start and end of stimulation. They respond to a variety of frequencies of stimulation ranging from 0.3 Hz to 3 Hz (Merkel's receptor), 3 Hz to 40 Hz (Meissner's corpuscle), 15 Hz to 400 Hz (Ruffini's cylinder), and 10 Hz to 500 Hz (pacinian corpuscle). So, all four mechanoreceptors would respond to slow rolling or massage with Ruffini's cylinders, and pacinian corpuscles also respond to high-frequency vibrations from machinery. Their major responsibilities are for proprioception so they would not play a major role in neural inhibition; however, Ruffini's and pacinian corpuscles may be able to contribute to the inhibition of sympathetic activity (contribute to muscle relaxation) (24). Ruffini's corpuscles are more sensitive to tangential forces and lateral stretch (25), which would be prominent with rolling, and their stimulation may decrease sympathetic nervous system activity (26). Perhaps the increased relaxation and decreases in heart rate and blood pressure with massage can be partially attributed to contributions from manual stimulation of Ruffini's and pacinian corpuscles (10).

Another series of receptors that can affect sympathetic and parasympathetic activation are the interstitial type III and IV receptors. These receptors have both low- and high-threshold sensory capabilities. They are more numerous than type I and II receptors, with both either having a thin myelinated sheath or being unmyelinated and originating from free nerve endings. They are multi-modal receptors (many functions) responding to pain, but also act as mechanoreceptors responding to tension and pressure. Their response to rapid and sustained pressure can contribute to decreases in heart rate, blood pressure, and ventilation, and lead to vasodilatation (27). Thus, they can also contribute to a more relaxed muscle with less resistance to a full range of movement.

There is growing evidence that mechanisms of rolling may be due more to the aforementioned neural as well as psychological mechanisms, rather than musculotendinous or myofascial factors. Magnusson et al. (28) have proposed that the acute or immediate increase in ROM after stretching is due to an increased stretch tolerance. In other words, while stretching the individual feels discomfort or pain, and the act of holding that position allows him or her to diminish or accommodate the painful or uncomfortable sensation. If the same muscle length or joint range of motion feels more tolerable then the person should be able to push themselves to an even greater range of motion. There could be both psychological and neural components to this effect.

Rolling can diminish different types of pain. Two studies from our lab punished participants with 10 sets of 10 squat repetitions. The objective was to induce delayed-onset muscle soreness (DOMS). In one study, participants were tested 24 and 48 hours after the squat protocol (6), whereas in the other they were also tested at 72 hours post-exercise (4). One of the groups would and the other would not roll before testing. In both studies, pain perception decreased when rolling was included post-exercise. DOMS-induced decreases in performance measures such as muscle activation, vertical jump, sprint time, and strength endurance were attenuated (less impairments) with rolling. So, was pain decreased because of self-myofascial release or central (neural) mechanisms? Subsequent rolling and pain studies from our lab illustrate the importance of the neural component.

Whereas DOMS pain may endure for up to 7 days due to muscle damage and inflammatory responses (29), muscle tender points may persist for weeks and months. Based on the aforementioned studies, rolling can inhibit short duration pain (DOMS), but does it have an effect on chronic pain (i.e. muscle tender points or trigger points)? A study by Aboodarda et al. (1) had a massage therapist identify the most sensitive muscle tender point on participants' plantar flexors (calf). Then the calf was massaged by the therapist, rolled, or not touched (control). One more condition was included which involved rolling of the contralateral calf. Both massaging and rolling the affected calf decreased the pain sensitivity of the muscle tender point. But even more interesting was that rolling the contralateral calf – no need to even touch the painful calf – reduced the pain sensitivity as well. In a similar study (30), we induced pain by electrically stimulating the tibial nerve of the plantar flexors with maximal and submaximal (70% of maximal current) intensity, high-frequency (50 Hz) electrical stimulation (tetanus). The experiment was not much fun for the participants because it involved maximal tolerable pain. Again, we rolled the affected calf, did nothing (control), or rolled the contralateral calf. Although each session of muscle stimulation increased pain sensitivity by about 10%, rolling the affected or contralateral calf inhibited the pain increase. Thus, if there is no need to touch the affected muscle and rolling another muscle decreases pain, then it is evident that some global neural response has occurred to decrease pain under chronic (muscle tender points), short-term (DOMS), and acute (tetanic stimulation) pain conditions.

In the aforementioned paper by Aboodarda et al. (1) pain depression occurred after light rolling massage. Nociceptors (pain receptors) are present in both muscle and skin (31,32) and thus even light rolling can increase the sensitivity of superficial nociceptors. Related to this finding, another study from our laboratory (33) reported that the intensity of rolling did not differentially affect the ROM, i.e. whether the roller massage was at 50%, 70%, or 90% of the maximum point of discomfort, the increase in ROM was similar.

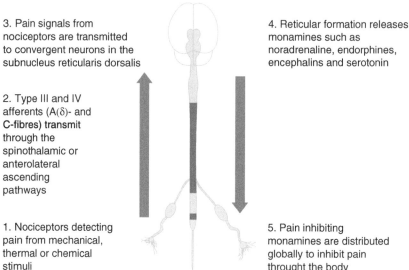

3. Pain signals from nociceptors are transmitted to convergent neurons in the subnucleus reticularis dorsalis

4. Reticular formation releases monamines such as noradrenaline, endorphines, encephalins and serotonin

2. Type III and IV afferents (A(δ)- and C-fibres) transmit through the spinothalamic or anterolateral ascending pathways

1. Nociceptors detecting pain from mechanical, thermal or chemical stimuli

5. Pain inhibiting monamines are distributed globally to inhibit pain throught the body

FIGURE 10.2 Diffuse noxious inhibitory control

There are a number of central nervous system possibilities including the gate control theory of pain (see Figure 8.7 in Chapter 8) (34,35), diffuse noxious inhibitory control (DNIC – Figure 10.2) (36), and parasympathetic nervous system alterations. The gate control theory of pain is commonly exemplified by somebody hurting a body part, and immediately grabbing and rubbing that same body part to minimize the pain. This action would stimulate many receptors and afferents, which would then be filtered at the brain. More technically the gate control theory involves activation of thick myelinated ergoreceptor (group III and IV afferents) nerve fibres (via activation of percutaneous [skin] and muscle mechanoreceptors, metaboreceptors, and proprioceptors) that modify the signals from ascending nociceptors (pain receptors) via small-diameter Aδ-fibres to the periaqueductal grey nucleus (35). Analgesia (pain suppression) then results from descending signals to opioid receptors, which would inhibit pain with serotoninergic and noradrenergic neurons (37).

Diffuse noxious inhibitory control, also known as counter-irritation, can be activated by nociceptive stimuli (i.e. mechanical pressure) from a non-local tissue. The typical practical application is that, if you banged your head against the cupboard, you can stub (hurt) your toe and the head pain would subjectively decrease. With DNIC, activation of non-local receptors is transmitted to multi-receptive convergent neurons, with a wide dynamic range, in the cortical subnucleus reticularis dorsalis, where it inhibits pain transmission monoaminergically (i.e. using monoamine transmitters such as noradrenaline and serotonin), reducing pain perception not only locally but also at distant sites (36–38).

Massage can also stimulate parasympathetic activation, with changes in serotonin, cortisol, endorphin, and oxytocin contributing to a decreased pain perception (10). Decreased parasympathetic reflexes could decrease pain sensitivity by reducing stress from myofascial tissue through relaxation of the strain on the smooth muscles embedded in the soft tissue. Massaging or rolling the muscle can produce acute ischaemic compression, which has been shown to result in reduced perceived pain in the upper trapezius muscles (39), and neck and shoulder muscles (40).

Massage decreases the afferent excitability of the α-motoneurons. A study from our laboratory found that both tapotement and pettrisage massage (41), as well as roller massage techniques, attenuated the Hoffmann (H)-reflex to muscle action potential (M)-wave ratio. Normalizing the H-reflex to the M-wave is an important technical procedure to ensure that any changes in the H-reflex are not due to alterations in the muscle's membrane action potential, but are actually due to changes in the afferent excitability of the motoneuron. The suppression of the spinal reflex excitability with the H-reflex may be attributed to decreased α-motoneuron excitability and/or increased presynaptic inhibition. A number of other studies have reported H-reflex inhibition with stretching (42–46) as well as massage (47,48). Massage has suppressed the H-reflex by 40–90% in these studies.

Thus, although ROM increases with massage and rolling may be attributed to thixotropic factors – a greater tolerance to the discomfort associated with musculotendinous lengthening (stretch tolerance) – there could also be reflexive inhibition decreasing stretch-induced contractile activity, resulting in a more relaxed muscle. Whether massage and rolling actually free myofascial restrictions is contentious due to the high forces that are needed, but more research is necessary to solidify this possible mechanism.

Rolling recommendations

What intensity and duration of rolling are optimal to achieve the greatest increases in ROM? Studies have demonstrated increased joint ROM with as little as 5–10 s of rolling, with 10 s providing significantly greater increases than 5 s (7). Most studies use multiple sets of 30- to 60-s bouts of rolling and, although not directly compared 60 s of rolling seem to provide further ROM improvements (2–6). However, in one study, 60, 90, and 120 s of rolling were applied between four sets of knee extensions. Although 120 s of rolling decreased the number of knee extension repetitions by 14%, the 90 and 60 s of rolling also decreased repetition numbers by 8–9% (49). This was one of the few studies that had reported impairments with rolling. As mentioned previously, whether rolling was conducted at 5, 7, or 9/10 on a pain scale, the increases in ROM were similar (33). Thus, there is no need to apply excruciating pain to achieve the desired results. Furthermore, following a typical warm-up (5 minutes of aerobic activity, static and dynamic stretching, and sport-specific activities), if rolling is performed at 10-minute intervals after the warm-up, the augmented ROM is maintained for 30 minutes to a greater degree than without intermittent rolling (50). This finding would be very important for those athletes who do not start a game or match and must sit on a bench for 10–30 minutes before entering the game. Continuing to roll while waiting on the bench would help maintain some of the benefits of the warm-up.

Vibration effects on ROM and performance

Local muscle vibration alone, and combined with static stretching, has been used to enhance ROM improvements. Vibration (35 Hz with 2-mm amplitude displacement) and static stretching have increased hamstring flexibility more than static stretching (7.8%) alone (51), whereas the combination has also improved the ability of male gymnasts to perform the forward splits (52). Local vibration (30 Hz at 4-mm displacement) alone demonstrated similar ROM increases to static stretching, with better results than dynamic stretching and whole-body vibration (53). There were no statistically significant differences compared with static stretching, but local vibration-induced ROM was consistently higher with magnitudes of a moderate effect. The vibration effects were especially effective with the most flexible participants (53). Another study also showed similar increases in ROM when comparing static stretching with vibration and static stretching combined (54). Finally, with synchronized swimmers, vibration (30 Hz at 2-mm displacement) improved passive but not active ROM (55). An early study (1976) used 15 minutes of vibrations to the low back and hamstrings (44 Hz with 0.1-mm displacements) and reported similar increases in ROM as static stretching (56). Their vibration displacement was very small, which could have been the difference between their study and other studies that did show a greater benefit with vibration.

Although the improved flexibility with vibration is relatively consistent, research reports on its effect on subsequent performance are mixed. Vibration has counteracted static stretch-induced impairments in jump height (57), and knee flexor and extensor forces (51), in two studies, but demonstrated that vibration alone or in combination with static stretching still induced impairments in strength and activation (54,58) in two other studies.

The mechanisms underlying the increased ROM with vibration have been attributed to a myriad of factors (55), including increased stretch (pain) threshold, increased blood flow associated with an increase in temperature, or vibration stress (59,60), which would decrease muscle viscosity and reduce the resistance to muscle extensibility. Vibration-induced muscle relaxation (61,62), and decreases in the phasic and static stretch reflexes (63) have also been reported. With even greater nuance, high-frequency (90 Hz) vibration affected short-latency responses more than medium-latency responses, but, when the vibration frequency was reduced to 30 Hz, there was a negligible effect on the short-latency reflex, although the medium-latency reflex was significantly reduced (64). Bove and colleagues (65) suggested that these effects were due to pre-synaptic inhibition of the group Ia afferent fibres or a gate control type limitation, where both vibration and stretching influence the same Ia pathways. Furthermore, if the stress were high enough, the combination of a strong stretch stimulus and substantial vibration could activate GTO inhibition through the Ib pathways (autogenic inhibition). However, GTO inhibition persists for only less than a second after the stimulus has been removed. In addition, other factors might include intrafusal fibre fatigue or persistence of motoneuron after-discharge due to reverberation of the interneuron pool (66).

So, addition of vibration to the stretching routine is probably not necessary for the average individual interested in improving this musculoskeletal health factor (flexibility), because stretching on its own should accomplish that objective. However, for those individuals who need to go further and achieve more extreme ROM, then vibration in concert with stretching might be recommended.

Summary

Whereas massage has been used for millennia, foam rollers and roller massagers have enjoyed recent popularity. Rolling can increase flexibility for approximately 20 minutes without subsequent performance deficits. Mechanisms underlying these ROM changes may be ascribed to decreased viscoelasticity (thixotropic effects), rolling-induced decreases in sympathetic activity and motoneuron excitability, and increased stretch tolerance. It is recommended to perform multiple sets of 30–60 seconds of rolling, which can be performed below the maximum pain tolerance (50–90% of maximum pain tolerance). Rolling may be combined with static stretching to further enhance ROM as well as applied at 10 minutes after the warm-up to maintain the increased flexibility achieved by this. Local muscle vibration can also increase ROM by increasing blood flow to the area, and decreasing viscoelasticity and reflex-induced neural inhibition, which may improve muscle relaxation.

Illustrative examples of rolling exercises for specific muscle groups

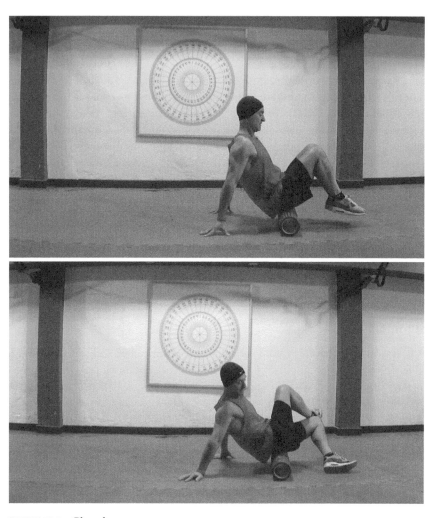

FIGURE 10.3 Gluteals

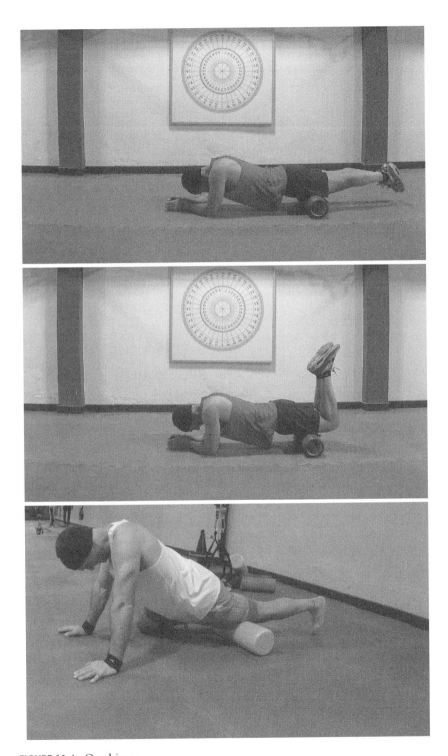

FIGURE 10.4 Quadriceps

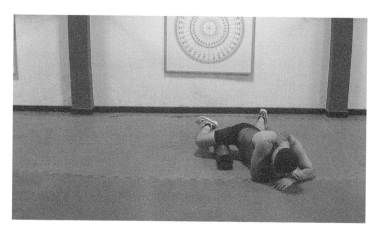

FIGURE 10.5 Adductors (groin)

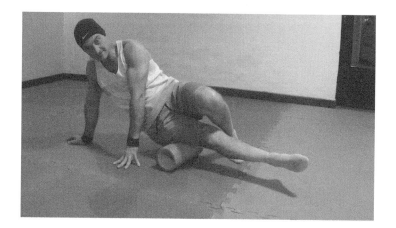

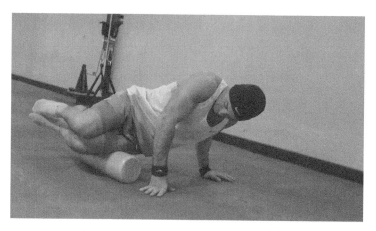

FIGURE 10.6 Tensor fascia latae

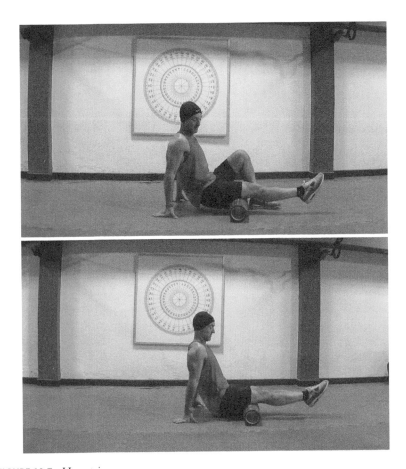

FIGURE 10.7 Hamstrings

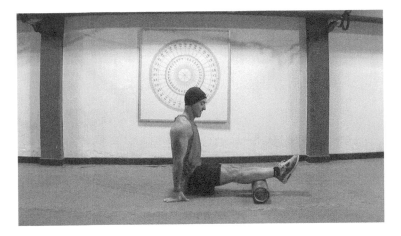

FIGURE 10.8 Plantar flexors

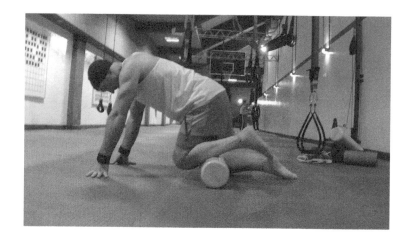

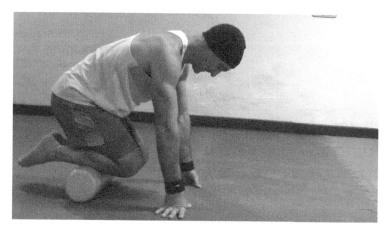

FIGURE 10.9 Tibialis anterior

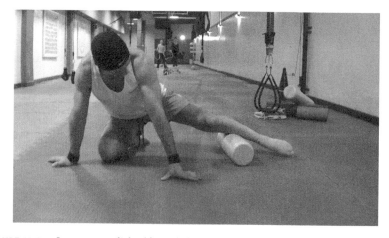

FIGURE 10.10 Inner or medial calf (medial soleus and gastrocnemius)

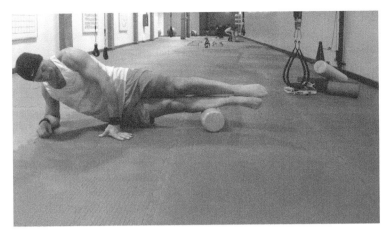

FIGURE 10.11   Outer or lateral calf (lateral soleus, gastrocnemius, and peronei)

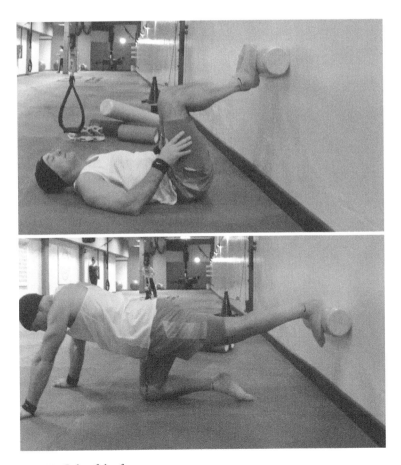

FIGURE 10.12   Sole of the foot

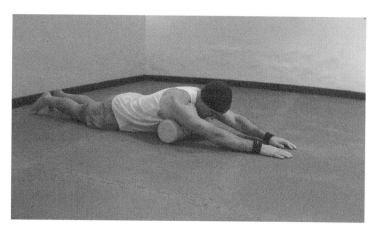

FIGURE 10.13 Pectorals

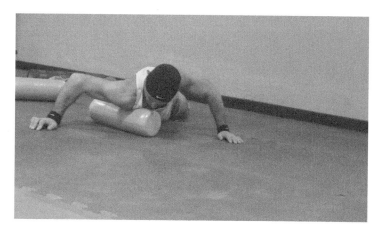

FIGURE 10.14 Pectorals and anterior deltoid

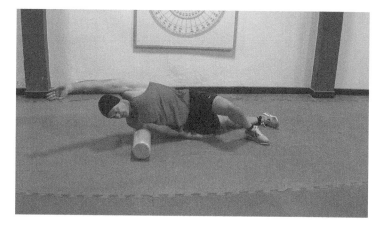

FIGURE 10.15 Lateral shoulder (deltoid) and arm (biceps and triceps brachii)

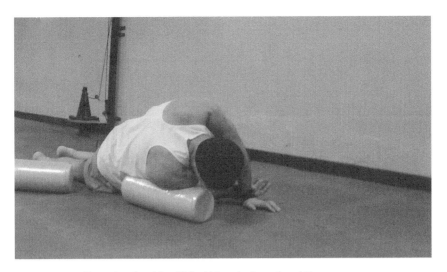

FIGURE 10.16 Posterior shoulder (deltoids) and triceps brachii

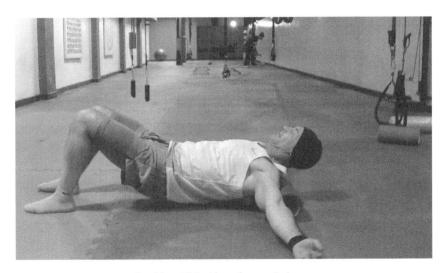

FIGURE 10.17 Posterior shoulders (deltoids and trapezius)

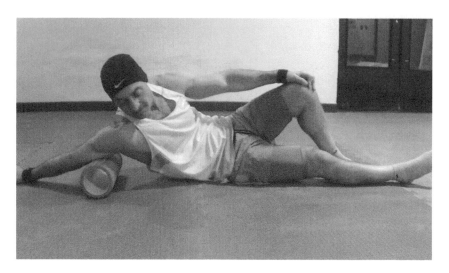

FIGURE 10.18 Biceps brachii

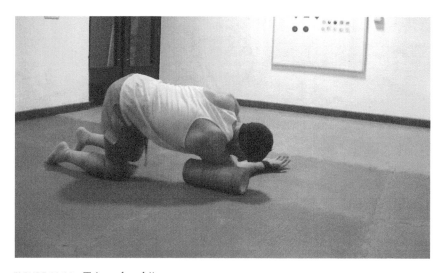

FIGURE 10.19 Triceps brachii

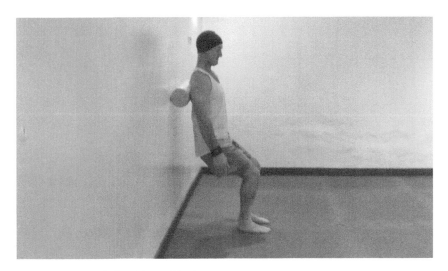

FIGURE 10.20 Back (upright position)

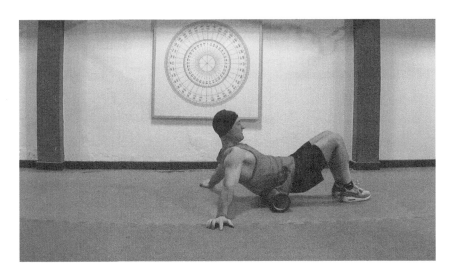

FIGURE 10.21 Lower back

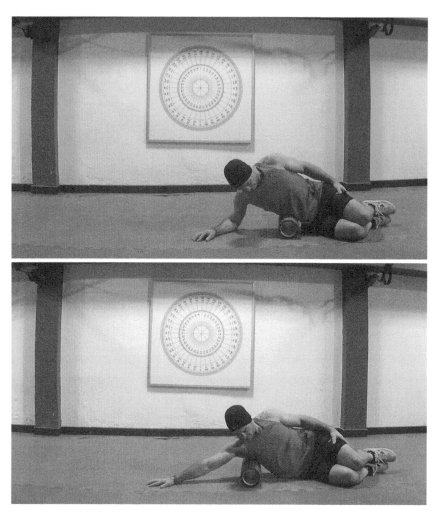

FIGURE 10.22 Lateral trunk

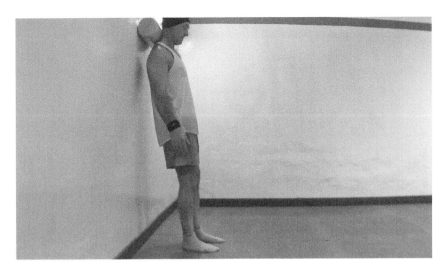

FIGURE 10.23   Neck

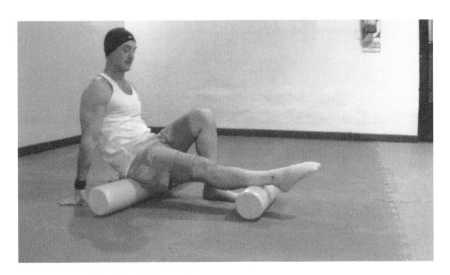

FIGURE 10.24   Gluteals and plantar flexors

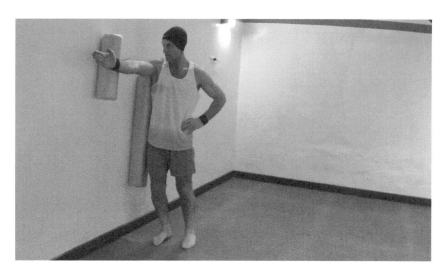

FIGURE 10.25   Back and arm

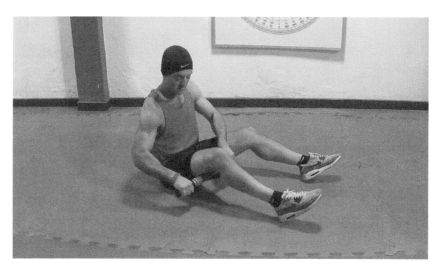

FIGURE 10.26   Roller massage of the hamstrings

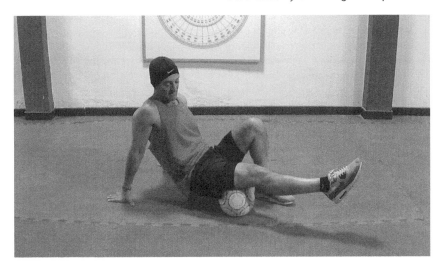

FIGURE 10.27 Exercise balls

References

1. Aboodarda SJ, Spence AJ, and Button DC. Pain pressure threshold of a muscle tender spot increases following local and non-local rolling massage. *BMC Musculoskelet Disord* 16: 265, 2015.
2. Bradbury-Squires DJ, Noftall JC, Sullivan KM, Behm DG, Power KE, and Button DC. Roller-massager application to the quadriceps and knee-joint range of motion and neuromuscular efficiency during a lunge. *J Athl Train* 50: 133–140, 2015.
3. Halperin I, Aboodarda SJ, Button DC, Andersen LL, and Behm DG. Roller massager improves range of motion of plantar flexor muscles without subsequent decreases in force parameters. *Int J Sports Phys Ther* 9: 92–102, 2014.
4. Macdonald GZ, Button DC, Drinkwater EJ, and Behm DG. Foam rolling as a recovery tool after an intense bout of physical activity. *Med Sci Sports Exerc* 46: 131–142, 2014.
5. MacDonald GZ, Penney MD, Mullaley ME, Cuconato AL, Drake CD, Behm DG, and Button DC. An acute bout of self-myofascial release increases range of motion without a subsequent decrease in muscle activation or force. *J Strength Cond Res* 27: 812–821, 2013.
6. Pearcey GE, Bradbury-Squires DJ, Kawamoto JE, Drinkwater EJ, Behm DG, and Button DC. Foam rolling for delayed-onset muscle soreness and recovery of dynamic performance measures. *J Athl Train* 50: 5–13, 2015.
7. Sullivan KM, Silvey DB, Button DC, and Behm DG. Roller-massager application to the hamstrings increases sit-and-reach range of motion within five to ten seconds without performance impairments. *Int J Sports Phys Ther* 8: 228–236, 2013.
8. Schleip R. Fascial plasticity – A new neurobiological explanation: Part 2. *J Bodyw Mov Ther* 7: 104–116, 2003.
9. Schleip R. Fascial plasticity – A new neurobiological explanation: Part I. *J Bodyw Mov Ther* 7: 11–19, 2003.

10. Weerapong P, Hume PA, and Kolt GS. The mechanisms of massage and effects on performance, muscle recovery and injury prevention. *Sports Med* 35: 235–256, 2005.
11. Skarabot J, Beardsley C, and Stirn I. Comparing the effects of self-myofascial release with static stretching on ankle range-of-motion in adolescent athletes. *Int J Sports Phys Ther* 10: 203–212, 2015.
12. Junker DH and Stoggl TL. The foam roll as a tool to improve hamstring flexibility. *J Strength Cond Res* 29: 3480–3485, 2015.
13. Kelly S and Beardsley C. Specific and cross-over effects of foam rolling on ankle dorsiflexion range of motion. *Int J Sports Phys Ther* 11: 544–551, 2016.
14. Mohr AR, Long BC, and Goad CL. Effect of foam rolling and static stretching on passive hip-flexion range of motion. *J Sport Rehabil* 23: 296–299, 2014.
15. Grieve R, Goodwin F, Alfaki M, Bourton AJ, Jeffries C, and Scott H. The immediate effect of bilateral self myofascial release on the plantar surface of the feet on hamstring and lumbar spine flexibility: A pilot randomised controlled trial. *J Bodyw Mov Ther* 19: 544–552, 2015.
16. Behm DG, Blazevich AJ, Kay AD, and McHugh M. Acute effects of muscle stretching on physical performance, range of motion, and injury incidence in healthy active individuals: A systematic review. *Appl Physiol Nutr Metab* 41: 1–11, 2016.
17. Behm DG and Chaouachi A. A review of the acute effects of static and dynamic stretching on performance. *Eur J Appl Physiol* 111: 2633–2651, 2011.
18. Beardsley C and Skarabot J. Effects of self-myofascial release: A systematic review. *J Bodyw Mov Ther* 19: 747–758, 2015.
19. Behara B and Jacobson BH. The acute effects of deep tissue foam rolling and dynamic stretching on muscular strength, power, and flexibility in division i linemen. *J Strength Cond Res* 31 (4): 888–892, 2017.
20. Healey KC, Hatfield DL, Blanpied P, Dorfman LR, and Riebe D. The effects of myofascial release with foam rolling on performance. *J Strength Cond Res* 28: 61–68, 2014.
21. Mikesky AE, Bahamonde RE, Stanton K, Alvey T, and Fitton T. Acute effects of the stick on strength, power, and flexibility. *J Strength Cond Res* 16: 446–450, 2002.
22. Huang SY, Di Santo M, Wadden KP, Cappa DF, Alkanani T, and Behm DG. Short-duration massage at the hamstrings musculotendinous junction induces greater range of motion. *J Strength Cond Res* 24: 1917–1924, 2010.
23. Trajano GS, Nosaka K, and Blazevich AJ. Neurophysiological mechanisms underpinning stretch-induced force loss. *Sports Med* 47 (8): 1531–1541, 2017.
24. Wu G, Ekedahl R, Stark B, Carlstedt T, Nilsson B, and Hallin RG. Clustering of Pacinian corpuscle afferent fibres in the human median nerve. *Exp Brain Res* 126: 399–409, 1999.
25. Kruger L. *Cutaneous sensory system*. Boston, MA: Birkhauser, 1987.
26. Van Den Berg F and Cabri J. *Angewandte Physiologie – Das Bindegewebe des bewegungsapparates verstehen und beeinflussen*. Stuttgart, Germany: Georg Thième Verlag, 1999.
27. Mitchell JH and Schmidt RF. *Cardiovascular reflex control by afferent fibers from skeletal muscle receptors*. Bethesda, MA: American Physiological Society, 1977.
28. Magnusson SP, Simonsen EB, Aagaard P, Sorensen H, and Kjaer M. A mechanism for altered flexibility in human skeletal muscle. *J Physiol* 497 (Pt 1): 291–298, 1996.
29. Behm DG, Baker KM, Kelland R, and Lomond J. The effect of muscle damage on strength and fatigue deficits. *J Strength Cond Res* 15: 255–263, 2001.
30. Cavanaugh MT, Doweling A, Young JD, Quigley PJ, Hodgson DD, Whitten JH, Reid JC, Aboodarda SJ, and Behm DG. An acute session of roller massage prolongs voluntary

torque development and diminishes evoked pain. *Eur J Appl Physiol* 117 (1): 109–117, 2017.

31. Kosek E, Ekholm J, and Hansson P. Increased pressure pain sensibility in fibromyalgia patients is located deep to the skin but not restricted to muscle tissue. *Pain* 63: 335–339, 1995.

32. Kosek E, Ekholm J, and Hansson P. Pressure pain thresholds in different tissues in one body region. The influence of skin sensitivity in pressure algometry. *Scand J Rehabil Med* 31: 89–93, 1999.

33. Grabow L, Young JD, Alcock LR, Quigley PJ, Byrne JM, Granacher U, Skrabot J, and Behm DG. Higher quadriceps roller massage forces do not amplify range-of-motion increases or impair strength and jump performance. *J Strength Cond Res*, doi:10.1519/JSC.0000000000001906, 2018.

34. Melzack R and Wall PD. Pain mechanisms: A new theory. *Science* 150: 971–979, 1965.

35. Moayedi M and Davis KD. Theories of pain: From specificity to gate control. *J Neurophysiol* 109: 5–12, 2013.

36. Mense S. Neurobiological concepts of fibromyalgia – The possible role of descending spinal tracts. *Scand J Rheumatol Suppl* 113: 24–29, 2000.

37. Pud D, Granovsky Y, and Yarnitsky D. The methodology of experimentally induced diffuse noxious inhibitory control (DNIC)-like effect in humans. *Pain* 144: 16–19, 2009.

38. Sigurdsson A and Maixner W. Effects of experimental and clinical noxious counter-irritants on pain perception. *Pain* 57: 265–275, 1994.

39. Kostopoulos D, Nelson AJ, Jr., Ingber RS, and Larkin RW. Reduction of spontaneous electrical activity and pain perception of trigger points in the upper trapezius muscle through trigger point compression and passive stretching. *J Musculoskelet Pain* 16: 266–278, 2008.

40. Hanten WP, Olson SL, Butts NL, and Nowicki AL. Effectiveness of a home program of ischemic pressure followed by sustained stretch for treatment of myofascial trigger points. *Phys Ther* 80: 997–1003, 2000.

41. Behm DG, Peach A, Maddigan M, Aboodarda SJ, DiSanto MC, Button DC, and Maffiuletti NA. Massage and stretching reduce spinal reflex excitability without affecting twitch contractile properties. *J Electromyogr Kinesiol* 23: 1215–1221, 2013.

42. Avela J, Kyrilninen H, and Komi PV. Altered reflex sensitivity after repeated and prolonged passive muscle stretching. *J Appl Physiol* 86: 1283–1291, 1999.

43. Etnyre BR and Abraham LD. H-reflex changes during static stretching and two variations of proprioceptive neuromuscular facilitation techniques. *Electroencephalogr Clin Neurophysiol* 63: 174–179, 2005.

44. Guissard N and Duchateau J. Neural aspects of muscle stretching. *Exerc Sport Sci Rev* 34: 154–158, 2006.

45. Guissard N, Duchateau J, and Hainaut K. Muscle stretching and motoneuron excitability. *Eur J Appl Physiol* 58: 47–52, 1988.

46. Guissard N, Duchateau J, and Hainaut K. Mechanisms of decreased motoneurone excitation during passive muscle stretching. *Exp Brain Res* 137: 163–169, 2001.

47. Goldberg J, Sullivan SJ, and Seaborne DE. The effect of two intensities of massage on H-reflex amplitude. *Phys Ther* 72: 449–457, 1992.

48. Sullivan SJ, Williams LR, Seaborne DE, and Morelli M. Effects of massage on alpha motoneuron excitability. *Phys Ther* 71: 555–560, 1991.

49. Monteiro ER, Vigotsky A, Skarabot J, Brown AF, Del Melo Fiuza AGF, Gomes TM, Halperin I, and Da Silva Novaes J. Acute effects of different foam rolling volumes in the

interset rest period on maximum repetition performance. *Hong Kong Physiother J* 36: 57–62, 2017.

50. Hodgson DD, Quigley PJ, Whitten JHD, Reid JC, and Behm DG. Impact of 10-minute interval roller massage on performance and active range of motion. *J Strength Cond Res*, doi:10.1519/JSC.0000000000002271, 2017.

51. Jemni M, Mkaouer B, Marina M, Asllani A, and Sands WA. Acute static vibration-induced stretching enhanced muscle viscoelasticity but did not affect maximal voluntary contractions in footballers. *J Strength Cond Res* 28: 3105–3114, 2014.

52. Sands WA, McNeal JR, Stone MH, Russell EM, and Jemni M. Flexibility enhancement with vibration: Acute and long-term. *Med Sci Sports Exerc* 38: 720–725, 2006.

53. Kurt C. Alternative to traditional stretching methods for flexibility enhancement in well-trained combat athletes: Local vibration versus whole-body vibration. *Biol Sport* 32: 225–233, 2015.

54. Miller JD, Herda TJ, Trevino MA, and Mosier EM. The effects of passive stretching plus vibration on strength and activation of the plantar flexors. *Appl Physiol Nutr Metab* 41: 917–923, 2016.

55. Sands WA, McNeal JR, Stone MH, Kimmel WL, Haff GG, and Jemni M. The effect of vibration on active and passive range of motion in elite female synchronized swimmers. *Eur J Sport Sci* 8: 217–223, 2008.

56. Atha J and Wheatley DW. Joint mobility changes due to low frequency vibration and stretching exercise. *Br J Sports Med* 10: 26–34, 1976.

57. Fernandes IA, Kawchuk G, Bhambhani Y, and Gomes PS. Does vibration counteract the static stretch-induced deficit on muscle force development? *J Sci Med Sport* 16: 472–476, 2013.

58. Herda TJ, Ryan ED, Smith AE, Walter AA, Bemben MG, Stout JR, and Cramer JT. Acute effects of passive stretching vs vibration on the neuromuscular function of the plantar flexors. *Scand J Med Sci Sports* 19: 703–713, 2009.

59. Kerschan-Schindl K, Grampp S, Henk C, Resch H, Preisinger E, Fialka-Moser V, and Imhof H. Whole-body vibration exercise leads to alterations in muscle blood volume. *Clin Physiol* 21: 377–382, 2001.

60. Rittweger J, Beller G, and Felsenberg D. Acute physiological effects of exhaustive whole-body vibration exercise in man. *Clin Physiol* 20: 134–142, 2000.

61. Issurin VB, Liebermann DG, and Tenenbaum G. Effect of vibratory stimulation training on maximal force and flexibility. *J Sports Sci* 12: 561–566, 1994.

62. Van Den Tillaar R. Will whole-body vibration training help increase the range of motion of the hamstrings? *J Strength Cond Res* 20: 192–196, 2006.

63. Bishop B. Vibratory stimulation, Part I. Neurophysiology or motor responses evoked by vibratory stimulation. *Phys Ther* 54: 1273–1282, 1974.

64. Bove M, Nardone A, and Schieppati M. Effects of leg muscle tendon vibration on group Ia and group II reflex responses to stance perturbation in humans. *J Physiol* 550: 617–630, 2003.

65. Claus D, Mills KR, and Murray NM. The influence of vibration on the excitability of alpha motoneurones. *Electroencephalogr Clin Neurophysiol* 69: 431–436, 1988.

66. Bongiovanni LG and Hagbarth KE. Tonic vibration reflexes elicited during fatigue from maximal voluntary contractions in man. *J Physiol* 423: 1–14, 1990.

11

STRETCHING EXERCISE ILLUSTRATIONS

Contributions and photographs by James D. Young and Jonathan C. Reid

The following chapter provides photographs with explanations of a variety of stretching exercises that can be employed within a standard athletic warm-up or dedicated flexibility training sessions. A standardized warm-up is presented in Table 11.1, which outlines in general the allocation of flexibility, mobility, and activation activities.

TABLE 11.1 Standardized warm-up components – example

Submaximal aerobic warm-up	Static stretching	Mobility and activation	Dynamic stretching and sport-specific movements
Examples: running, jogging, bike (arms and legs), cycle ergometer, skipping, elliptical, attempt to increase core temperature by 1–2°C as evidenced by a sweating response	1–2 repetitions of 15–30 s per muscle group ($\leq$60 s per muscle group) 3–5 stretches Target restricted groups or relevant groups for training session	Choose 2 or 3 exercises to address weaknesses and 2–3 exercises for specific movement patterns, 5–8 repetitions per exercise Address common weaknesses or deficiencies (e.g. gluteal bridge, band hip flexor, banded lateral/forward walks, band pull-aparts Prepare movement patterns for workout (e.g. squat, hinge)	5–8 exercises, Example:10-m sprint out and back Elevate heart rate, prepare for workout, work on movement patterns
5–10 minutes	3–5 minutes maximum	3–6 minutes maximum	3-minute maximum

Static stretching exercise section

1. Lower body-stretching photos: quadriceps and hip flexors: Figures 11.1–11.4
2. Lower body-stretching photos: hamstrings: Figures 11.5–11.7
3. Lower body-stretching photos: gluteals: Figures 11.8–11.10
4. Lower body-stretching photos: groin adductors: Figure 11.11

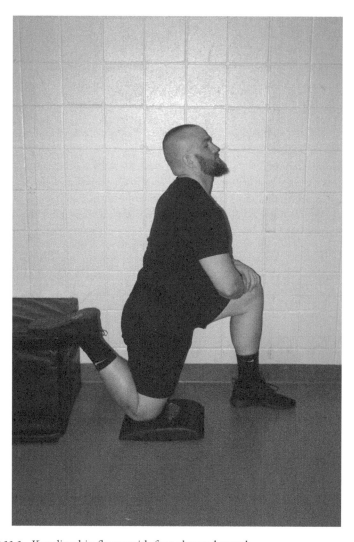

FIGURE 11.1 Kneeling hip flexor with foot elevated stretch

5. Lower body-stretching photos: calves (plantar flexors): Figures 11.12–11.14
6. Upper body-stretching photos: pectorals and latissimus dorsi: Figures 11.15–11.23
7. Upper body-stretching photos: neck: Figures 11.24–11.25

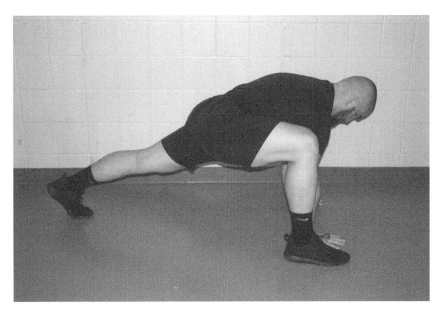

FIGURE 11.2 Forward lunge stretch with hand planted

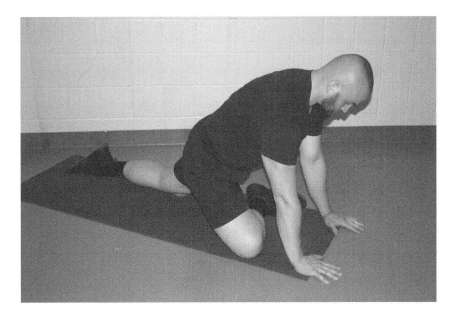

FIGURE 11.3 Pigeon stretch

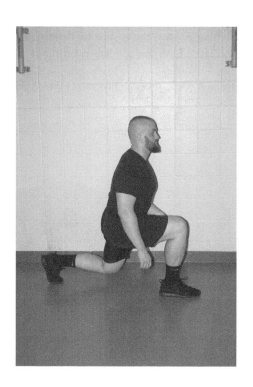

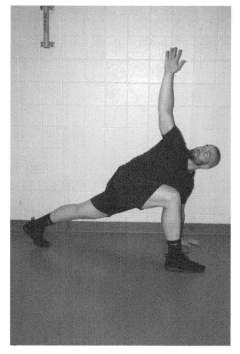

FIGURE 11.4 Lunge with a rotation

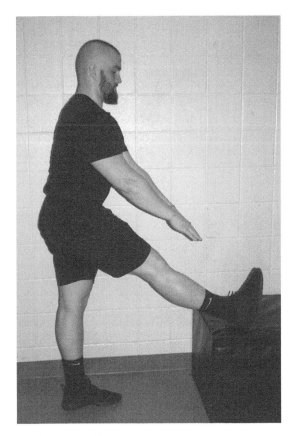

FIGURE 11.5 Single-leg elevated hamstring stretch

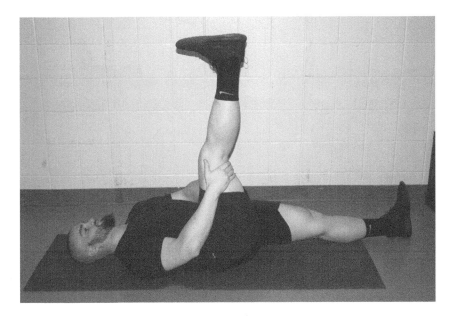

FIGURE 11.6 Supine single-leg hamstring stretch

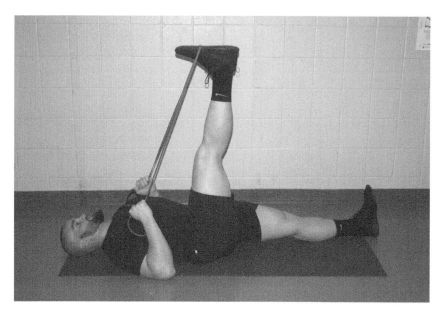

FIGURE 11.7   Band-assisted hamstring stretch

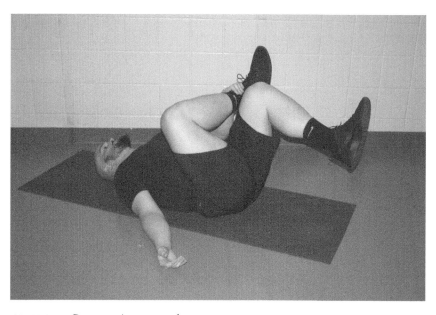

FIGURE 11.8   Reverse pigeon stretch

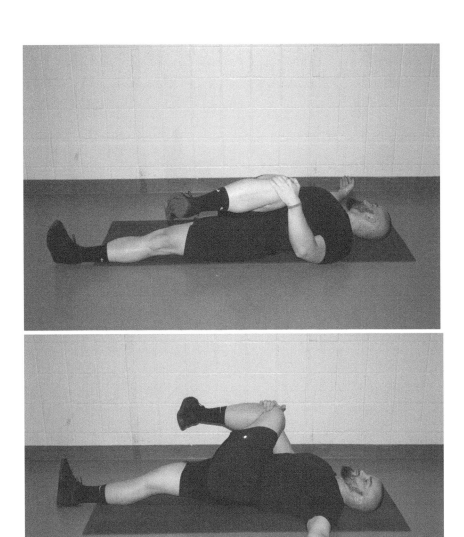

FIGURE 11.9 Supine single-leg rotation

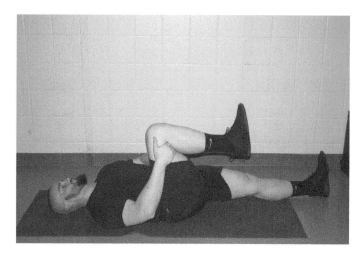

FIGURE 11.10 Lying hip flexion

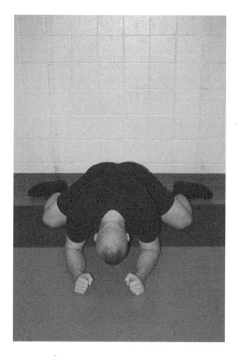

FIGURE 11.11 Adductor stretch

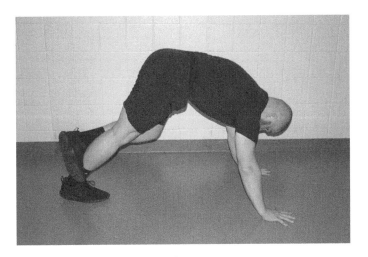

FIGURE 11.12 Push-up position calf stretch

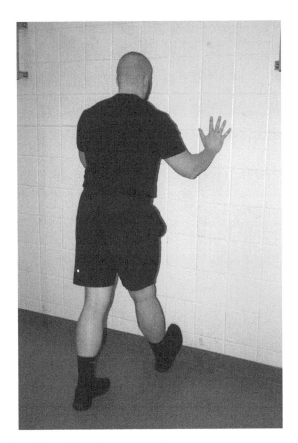

FIGURE 11.13 Standing calf stretch against wall

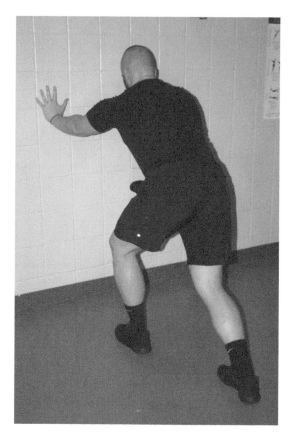

FIGURE 11.14 Standing soleus stretch

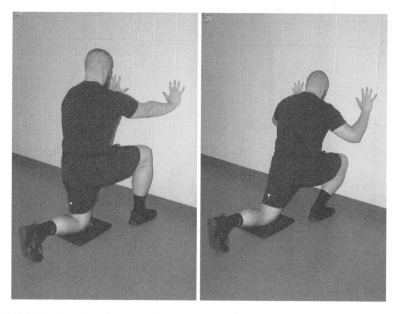

FIGURE 11.15 Kneeling lunge position soleus stretch

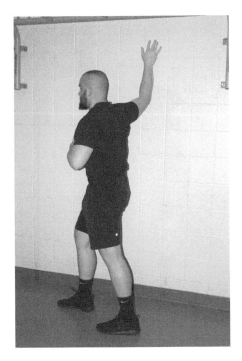

FIGURE 11.16   Pectoralis wall stretch with rotation

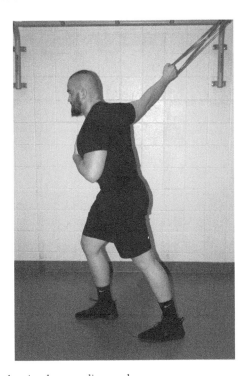

FIGURE 11.17   Band-assisted pectoralis stretch

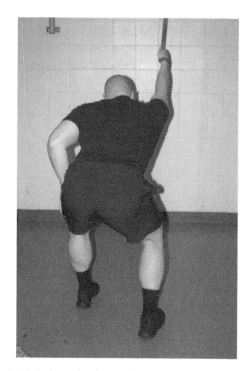

FIGURE 11.18 Banded latissimus dorsi stretch

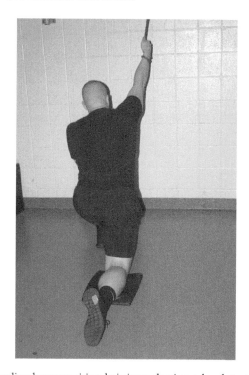

FIGURE 11.19 Kneeling lunge position latissimus dorsi overhead stretch

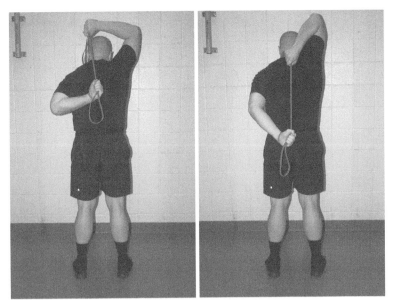

FIGURE 11.20   Triceps brachii and shoulder internal rotation band stretch

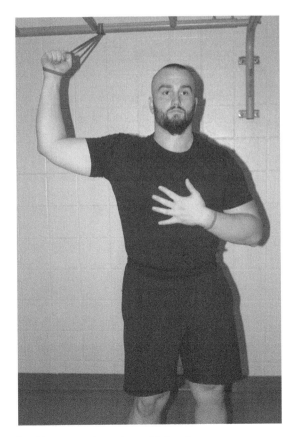

FIGURE 11.21   Shoulder external rotation with band

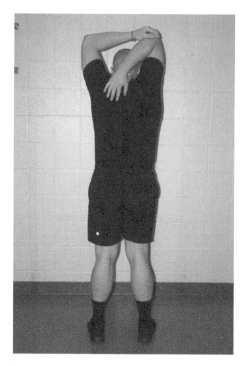

FIGURE 11.22   Overhead triceps brachii stretch

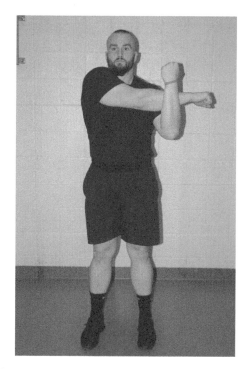

FIGURE 11.23   Deltoid cross-over stretch

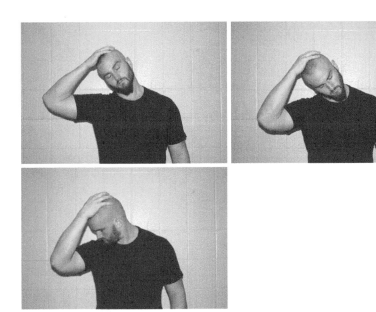

FIGURE 11.24 Neck series

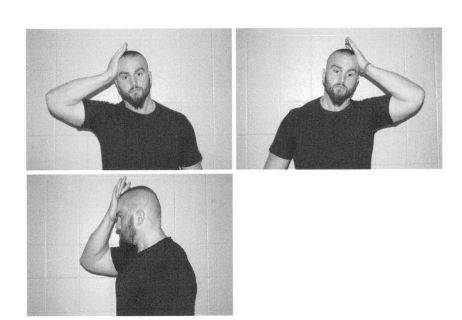

FIGURE 11.25 Neck-strengthening series

Mobility exercise section

1. Lower body mobility photos: Figures 11.26–11.39
2. Upper body mobility photos: Figures 11.40–11.47

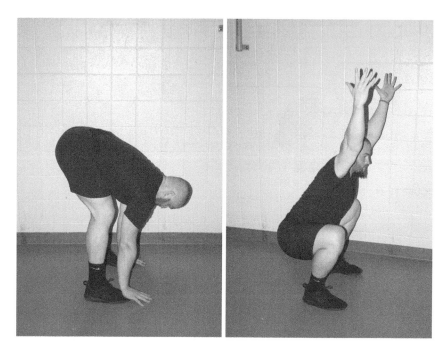

FIGURE 11.26 Hip mobility hinge and overhead squat sequence

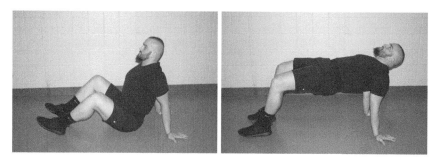

FIGURE 11.27 Dynamic hip bridge with arms extended

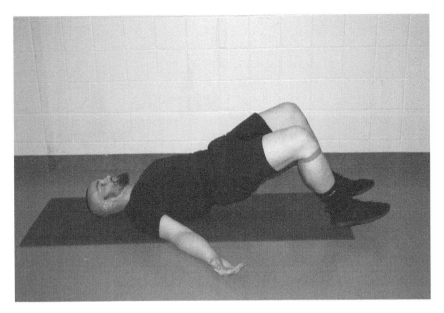

FIGURE 11.28 Dynamic hip bridge with band

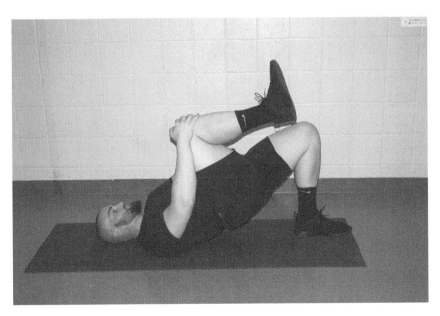

FIGURE 11.29 Dynamic alternating hip bridge with a knee-to-chest hold

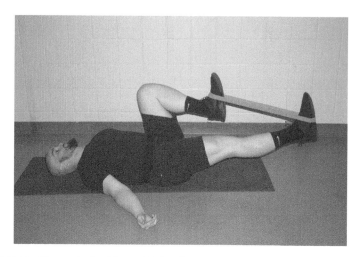

FIGURE 11.30 Dynamic dead bug with band

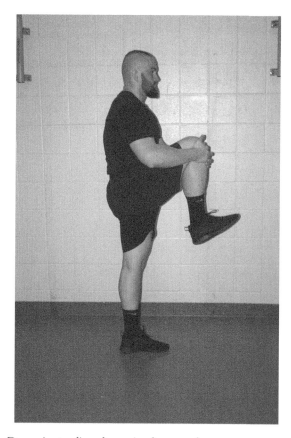

FIGURE 11.31 Dynamic standing alternating knee to chest

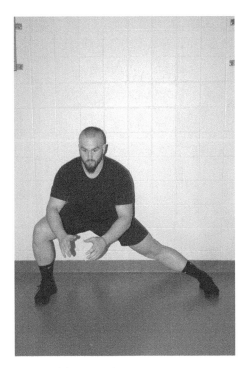

FIGURE 11.32 Dynamic lateral lunge with pause

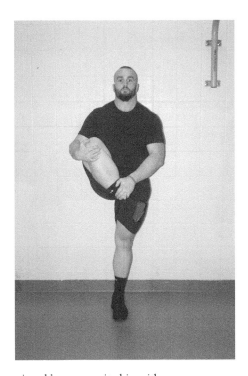

FIGURE 11.33 Dynamic ankle to opposite hip with pause

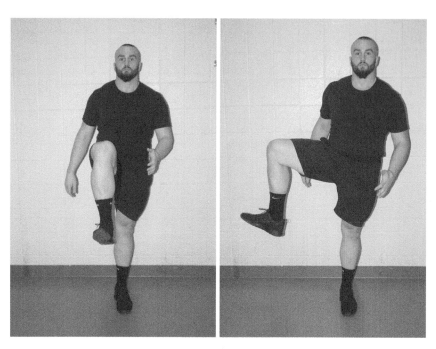

FIGURE 11.34 Dynamic external rotation of hip

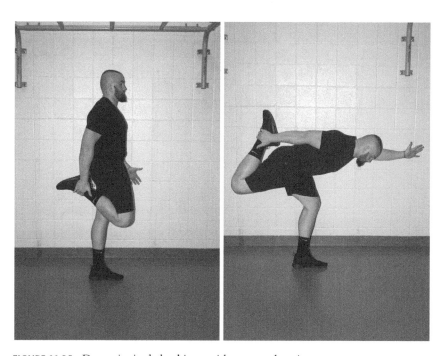

FIGURE 11.35 Dynamic single leg hinge with arm reach series

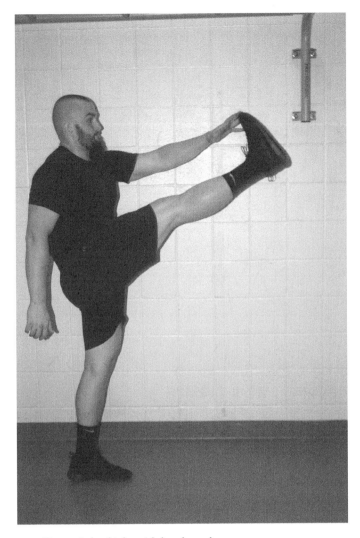

FIGURE 11.36 Dynamic leg kicks with hand touch

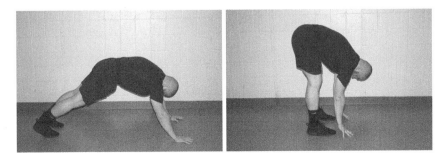

FIGURE 11.37 Dynamic inch worm with pause

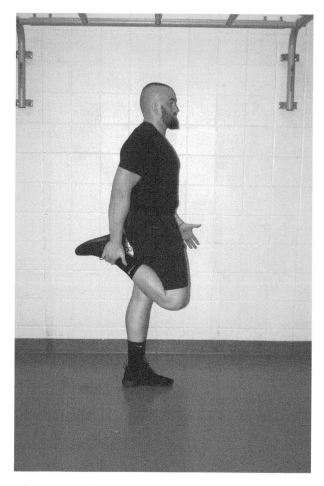

FIGURE 11.38 Dynamic quadriceps squeeze with a pause

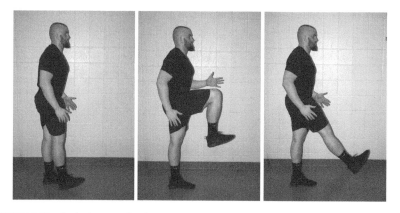

FIGURE 11.39 Sprinting mechanics

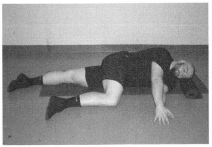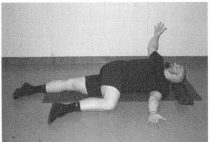

FIGURE 11.40 Side-lying rotation

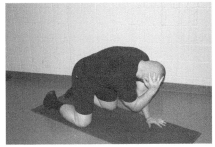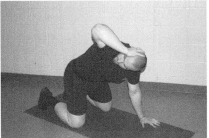

FIGURE 11.41 Kneeling dynamic rotation

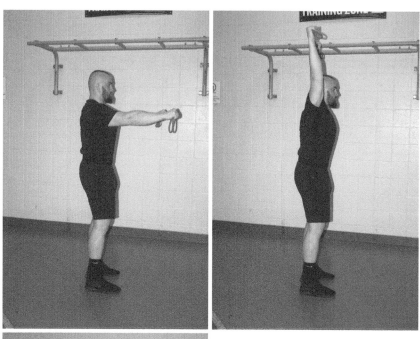

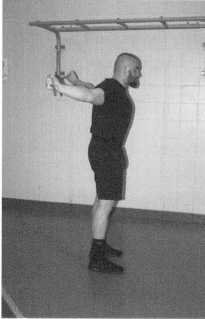

FIGURE 11.42 Dynamic band shoulder pullovers

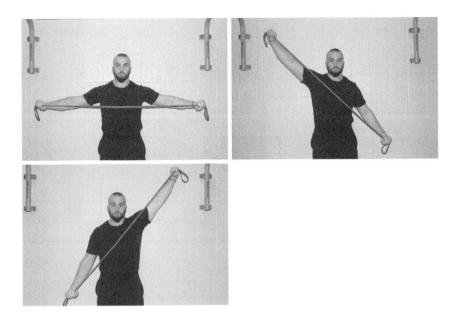

FIGURE 11.43 Band pull-apart series

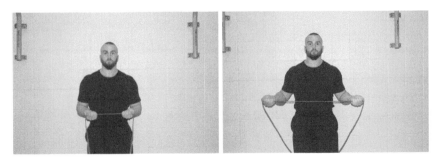

FIGURE 11.44 Band shoulder external rotation

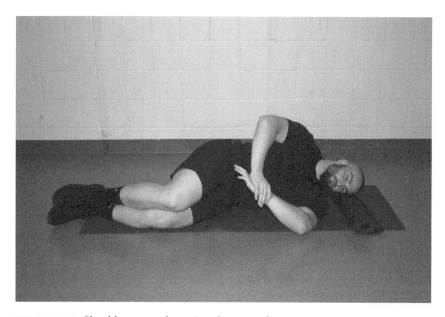

FIGURE 11.45 Shoulder external rotation sleep stretch

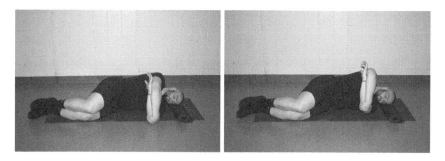

FIGURE 11.46 Scapular protraction sleep stretch: (a) start position; (b) end position

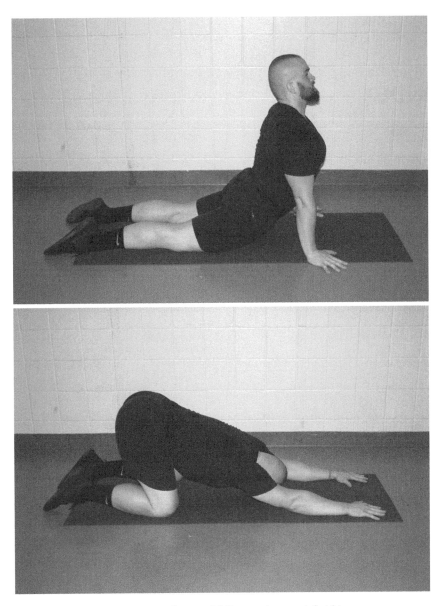

FIGURE 11.47 Dynamic prone cobra to child's pose (start and finish)

INDEX

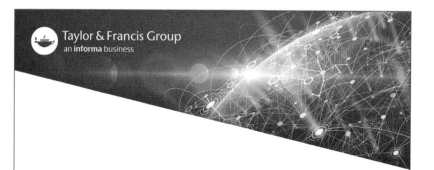